Dementia

YOUR QUESTIONS ANSWERED TION SERVICES

Commissioning Editor: Fiona Conn
Project Development Manager: Fiona Conn
Project Manager: Frances Affleck
Designer: George Ajayi

Dementia

YOUR QUESTIONS ANSWERED

Jeremy Brown
MA MD FRCP
Consultant Neurologist, Addenbrooke's Hospital, Cambridge, UK

Jonathan Hillam
BSc MBBS MRCPsych
Consultant in Old Age Psychiatry, The Julian Hospital, Norwich, UK

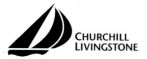

CHURCHILL
LIVINGSTONE

EDINBURGH LONDON NEW YORK OXFORD PHILADELPHIA ST LOUIS SYDNEY TORONTO 2004

CHURCHILL LIVINGSTONE
An imprint of Elsevier Science Limited

Cover image by kind permission of Dr Peter Johannsen, Dementia Clinic Aarhus University Hospital, Denmark.

Sample items from the Mini Mental State examination reproduced by permission of the publisher, Psychological Assessment Resources Inc. from the Mini Mental State Examination by Marshal Folstein and Susan Folstein © 1975, 1998, 2001 by Mini Mental LLC, Inc.

First published 2004

ISBN 0 4330 266 3

British Library Cataloguing in Publication Data
A catalogue record for this book is available from the British Library

Library of Congress Cataloging in Publication Data
A catalog record for this book is available from the Library of Congress

Notice
Medical knowledge is constantly changing. Standard safety precautions must be followed, but as new research and clinical experience broaden our knowledge, changes in treatment and drug therapy may become necessary or appropriate. Readers are advised to check the most current product information provided by the manufacturer of each drug to be administered to verify the recommended dose, the method and duration of administration, and contraindications. It is the responsibility of the practitioner, relying on experience and knowledge of the patient, to determine dosages and the best treatment for each individual patient. Neither the Publisher nor the authors assume any liability for any injury and/or damage to persons or property arising from this publication.
The Publisher

ELSEVIER SCIENCE
your source for books, journals and multimedia in the health sciences

www.elsevierhealth.com

The publisher's policy is to use **paper manufactured from sustainable forests**

Printed in China

Contents

To Lucy, Billy, Jessie, Theo and Molly; Claire, Poppy, Liberty and Jude.

Preface

Dementia, and dementia care, has for long been a neglected topic. However, the last decade has witnessed an explosion of interest in the condition not only from the scientific and medical communities but also from the general public. This is partly due to the perceived threat posed by the health needs of an ageing population. But there is also a new sense of therapeutic optimism brought on by the emergence of drugs aimed at delaying the decline of Alzheimer's disease. As a result there is now a greater understanding of dementia by health professionals, and care for patients and their carers is slowly improving.

Dementia is a syndrome – a cluster of symptoms – and not a diagnosis in its own right. Its causes are wide ranging, including not only primary degenerative and vascular disorders but also many other physical conditions. Symptoms are often diverse, encompassing psychiatric and neurological symptoms and behavioural changes as well as cognitive impairment. Dementia is, therefore, diagnostically challenging, and assessing and managing patients with dementia is a lengthy process. Small wonder that primary care health workers often feel they neither have the time nor the expertise to do so properly. Yet it is a common disorder. Although specialist services for dementia in the UK have grown dramatically over the last twenty years, such services can only assess and manage a small proportion of patients with dementia. Primary care therefore has an important role to play; not only in identifying and diagnosing patients with dementia and other memory disorders, but also by remaining involved as the disease progresses. It is not just patients who need this contact: spouses, carers and other involved family members are also 'sufferers', and advice, information, and practical and emotional support can make a real difference during the difficult years ahead. Such help has been shown to delay placement into residential care and reduce psychological morbidity experienced by carers

Dementia: Your Questions Answered has been written with a wide readership in mind. It will provide primary care workers – doctors, nurses, and other clinical staff – with the information they need to give patients and carers the support they deserve. It is not intended to be a comprehensive textbook on dementia: instead it aims to answer questions which – the authors believe – non-specialist clinicians might ask, or be asked, when faced with a patient or carer in clinic, or when confronted by a report written by a specialist. It will also be useful to clinical staff working with patients with dementia in other settings such as psychiatric and geriatric wards, and residential homes. Moreover, the book provides much relevant and accessible information to non-medical readers, particularly carers.

JB
JH

Acknowledgements

JB would like to thank Dr Sian Thompson for her careful reading of the manuscript.

JH wishes to thank the general practitioners in West Norfolk whose questions, suggestions and comments greatly helped in the preparation of the book.

JB
JH

How to use this book

The *Your Questions Answered* series aims to meet the information needs of GPs and other primary care professionals who care for patients with chronic conditions. It is designed to help them work with patients and their families, providing effective, evidence-based care and management.

The books are in an accessible question and answer format, with detailed contents lists at the beginning of every chapter and a complete index to help find specific information.

ICONS

Icons are used in the book to identify particular types of information:

 highlights information important to clinical practice

 highlights side effect information

 highlights case studies which illustrate or help to explain the answers given

PATIENT QUESTIONS

At the end of relevant chapters there are sections of frequently asked patient questions, with easy-to-understand answers aimed at the non-medical reader. These questions are also listed at the end of the book.

What is dementia?

1

DEFINITIONS AND CLASSIFICATION

1.1 How is dementia defined?

According to the International Classification of Diseases (ICD 10) (WHO 1992), dementia is defined as:

A syndrome due to disease of the brain, usually of a chronic or progressive nature in which there is disturbance of multiple higher cortical function including memory, thinking, orientation, comprehension, calculation, language and judgement. Consciousness is not clouded. The impairments of cognitive function are commonly accompanied, and occasionally preceded by deterioration in emotional control, social behaviour or motivation.

1.2 What is dementia not?

Although most definitions specify that dementia is a 'global' impairment, this is an oversimplification. However, any impairment will be sufficient to adversely affect an individual's daily functioning. A diagnosis of dementia should be made only if the cognitive symptoms and impairment have been present for at least 6 months. | What is DEMENTIA?

Dementia is a syndrome (i.e. it is not a single disease entity). It is acquired later in life and is usually, but not always, progressive. In most cases it is irreversible. This definition thereby distinguishes dementia from various superficially similar brain conditions such as delirium, learning disability, focal cerebral damage due to stroke and age-related memory loss.

There is some debate as to whether to classify the cognitive sequelae of reversible physical disorders as dementia. In most cases, the cognitive impairment is not progressive and usually resolves (although not always completely) on resolution of the causative condition. It is therefore vital to exclude any reversible 'causes of dementia' before diagnosing a degenerative or other irreversible condition. TYPES OF DEMENTIA

Different dementias affect different parts of the brain. Alzheimer's disease affects the parietal and temporal lobes whereas frontotemporal dementias affect the anterior temporal and frontal lobes (*Fig. 1.1*).

1.3 What is the difference between dementia and encephalopathy?

Encephalopathies and dementias are part of the same disease spectrum. A disease evolving over days to weeks is called an encephalopathy; one evolving over months to years a dementia. Encephalopathies, with their shorter history, are more amenable to treatment than long-standing dementias. Encephalopathies are more likely to be secondary to disease elsewhere in the body.

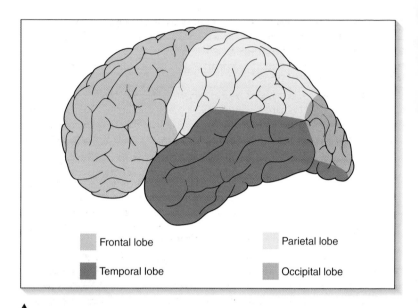

▲

Fig. 1.1 The lobes of the brain.

1.4 How are the types of dementia classified?

The ICD 10 classifies dementia as follows:

- dementia in Alzheimer's disease
- vascular dementia (and subtypes including subcortical vascular dementia)
- dementia in other diseases (e.g. Pick's disease, Parkinson's disease, Huntington's disease, Creutzfeldt–Jakob disease, HIV and in other specified diseases such as multiple sclerosis, metabolic disorders, vitamin B_{12} deficiency)
- unspecified dementia.

1.5 What about other types of dementia?

More subtypes of dementia have been described than those listed above. Although they are not specified in current diagnostic systems, they do appear to have clinical significance. An alternative classification could read as follows:

- Primary degenerative disorders (e.g. Alzheimer's disease, frontal lobe dementias including Pick's disease, dementia with Lewy bodies).
- Vascular dementias including variants such as Binswanger's disease.

■ Secondary dementias due to CNS or other systemic pathology, e.g. hydrocephalus, vitamin B$_{12}$ deficiency. Many dementias in this group could be reversible (see Chapter 4).

1.6 What is 'senile dementia'?

This term is now obsolete. It used to be applied to any patient suffering from dementia who also happened to be old. Conventionally, this has been taken to mean over the age of 65 years and many clinical services in the UK have been organized around this age 'cut off'. The use of 'senile dementia' reflected the fact that until recently there was little knowledge of, or interest in, the different causes of dementia in the elderly. Most were assumed to suffer from 'cerebral arteriosclerosis'. The diagnosis of Alzheimer's disease was reserved for younger patients with the disease. Older patients with similar symptoms were described as having 'Senile dementia – Alzheimer type' (SDAT).

1.7 What is 'benign senescent forgetfulness'?

It should be emphasized that dementia should not be diagnosed on memory loss alone; evidence of other forms of cognitive decline is also required. Many people become more forgetful as they get older. Recalling names, for example, is a particularly common difficulty. There are various terms for this, including 'benign senescent forgetfulness' and 'age-related cognitive decline'.

1.8 What is 'MCI'?

Other people develop more serious memory loss similar to that seen in patients with very mild Alzheimer's disease. This is often called 'mild cognitive impairment' (MCI). Not all patients with such conditions will develop dementia but the risk is greater than in the general population. Work is being undertaken to identify factors that will predict who is most at risk and to determine whether drugs given to patients with MCI might delay the onset of Alzheimer's disease.

Mild Cognitive Disorder is a specific diagnosis in ICD 10 that refers to objective and usually temporary cognitive impairment associated with a discrete physical disorder.

PREVALENCE OF DEMENTIA

1.9 How common is dementia?

The prevalence of dementia increases with age (*Table 1.1*). Findings from community studies in the UK vary somewhat but, overall, indicate that the prevalence of dementia at 70 years is between 2 and 7%. This rises to 25% beyond 85 years of age. There are around 800 000 dementia sufferers in the UK.

Statistics.

Table 1.1 Age-specific prevalence rates (per 100 population) for dementia in Europe				
Age range (years)				
31–60	**61–70**	**71–80**	**81–90**	**90+**
0.1	1.5	5.0	25	35

1.10 What is the age of onset of dementia?

The typical age of onset varies according to the type of dementia but in general it is uncommon before the fifth decade. On average, frontal lobe dementia has an earlier age of onset than Alzheimer's disease. Overall, in Europe and North America, Alzheimer's disease is the most common cause of dementia, with higher proportions of vascular dementia in Japan and China. Alzheimer's disease is slightly more common in women than in men, and vice versa for vascular dementia.

RISK FACTORS

1.11 Who is at risk of developing dementia?

The aetiology of the various types of dementia will be discussed later. However, a number of factors increase an individual's risk of developing dementia:

- A *strong* family history, i.e. an established dementia (particularly of early-onset Alzheimer's disease, or Huntington's disease) in a first-degree relative is a known risk factor.
- Prolonged hypertension, uncontrolled diabetes, atrial fibrillation or a history of transient ischaemic attacks or stroke are all risk factors for vascular dementias.
- Repeated head trauma is said to increase the risk of both Alzheimer's disease and dementia associated with Parkinsons's disease.
- More controversially, but supported by some compelling evidence, are the hypotheses that there is an association between chronic, late onset depression and dementia
- There is a causative link between exposure to prion proteins through human growth factor, corneal transplantation or the consumption of BSE-infected meat, and Creutzfeldt–Jakob disease.

1.12 Who is less at risk of developing dementia?

All things being equal, a high level of premorbid intellectual functioning – as measured, for example, by level of education attained and, specifically, verbal ability – is believed to reduce the risk of developing dementia. The risk might also be reduced in individuals who maintain a high level of mental activity into old age. It is possible that there is a protective effect in that such a person can withstand greater degrees of cerebral pathology before exhibiting signs of significant cognitive deficit.

1.13 Do patients who complain about their poor memory always have dementia?

It is often suggested that if you worry that you are developing dementia then you are probably not doing so. Some patients make persistent complaints about their poor memory. Often, there is little to find on objective cognitive testing. In these circumstances there is less likely to be any identifiable organic brain impairment – such complaints are more typically associated with anxiety and depression. However, recent studies suggest that older people with subjective memory complaints are between 2 and 4 times more likely to develop dementia subsequently.

1.14 Do patients realize that they are developing dementia?

Patients in the early stages of the condition might be aware of their declining memory and functional ability, and this can cause distress, anxiety or depression. However, this awareness is typically lost as the disease progresses, leading to a denial of the problems and, frequently, refusal of offers of help. Some forms of dementia, such as Alzheimer's disease and frontal lobe dementia, are associated with earlier loss of insight than other forms. Patients with early dementia might well agree, when asked, that their memory is impaired. However, they often play down the significance of this.

1.15 How can I tell whether a patient is 'worried well' or has the early stages of degenerative dementia?

Three quick guides are:

■ Ask for a history from someone else – usually a spouse/partner but sometimes a friend or work colleague. Patients with dementia tend to underestimate their own problems, do not usually initiate the consultation and have to be persuaded to come. Once in the consulting room, they let the spouse, friend or colleague take the dominant role. When asked about their memory, patients often admit that there are problems but feel that these are being exaggerated. If interviewed in the presence of the patient, a spouse might be restrained by loyalty but, given the appropriate chance, will often admit that there are very real problems.

■ Ask the patient or the spouse/partner to give you an example of when there has been a problem resulting from a memory lapse. It is then a matter of judging whether this is within the bounds of normality.

'Worried well' patients are often unable to give an example or will say that they forgot a dental appointment. An organic story is the grandfather who took his two young grandsons to a school football match and came back without them, and who later could not really understand what he had done wrong.

■ Ask for examples of skills lost.

1.16 What symptoms distinguish early Alzheimer's disease from the 'worried well'?

A number of symptoms occur in the early stages of Alzheimer's disease but also occur in many normal people. These symptoms can be organic and are not discriminatory. Examples are:

■ going upstairs and then forgetting why
■ going shopping and not buying all the required items
■ becoming lost on a half familiar route
■ forgetting dental appointments, etc.
■ failing to pass on telephone messages.

Other symptoms are strong indicators of organic disease:

■ repeating the same question several times in an evening
■ forgetting that conversations ever took place even when reminded
■ becoming lost in a familiar place
■ failing to remember new information, e.g. never learning where the loo is when staying in a hotel for a week.

Alzheimer's disease is rare below the age of 55 years. Many 'worried well' patients present between the ages of 35 and 55 years.

1.17 How does a 'worried well' patient behave?

Worried well patients are often seen in memory clinics. It is wise never to be too certain of the diagnosis early on. A number of patients appear to be worried well for a couple of years and then develop unmistakably organic problems. However, there is a distinctive pattern with worried well patients:

■ They come alone to the clinic – even if asked to come with a partner. If asked why they came alone they say that it isn't necessary to bother their wife/husband.
■ If asked whether their partner is concerned about their memory they say it is a bit of a family joke or that their husband says his own memory is just as bad (only men seem to say this!).
■ When asked if their memory lapses have led to complaints at work they explain that they manage to cover up their problems; they are often proud of their work performance.

Age alone is a good indicator of the likelihood of the patient having an organic dementia. Dementias are extremely rare below the age of 40 years. Patients presenting below the age of 55 years are likely to be 'worried well'; those presenting after 60 years are much more likely to have an early dementia.

1.18 Is there a more objective method of telling the 'worried well' from early Alzheimer's disease?

Rating scales provide a more objective assessment of a patient. These include the Mental Test Score (MTS), the Mini Mental State Examination (MMSE) and the Addenbrookes Cognitive Examination (ACE; see Appendix 1). The ACE includes the 30 points from the MMSE but also tests anterograde memory, verbal fluency and naming of line drawings, amongst a number of other tasks. It is scored out of a total of a 100; the average score is 94. Patients scoring above this level are unlikely to develop a degenerative dementia in the next 2 years. Patients with a score below 88 are at higher risk of developing a progressive dementia.

An overall score of less that 88 is suspicious of early Alzheimer's disease or some other form of dementia, although many normal patients have scores in this region. A score of less than 80 suggests a dementia or some educational or developmental problem.

DIFFERENTIAL DIAGNOSIS

1.19 What is delirium?

Delirium is a transiently altered mental state characterized by:

- fluctuating cognitive impairment
- rapid onset
- clouding of consciousness
- psychotic symptoms, typically visual hallucinations and paranoid delusions
- abnormalities of motor activity; both under- and overactivity occur
- emotional changes; fear, perplexity, etc.

1.20 What are the causes of delirium?

There are many causes. It can be due to bacterial or viral infection, electrolyte imbalance or metabolic abnormality. Poisoning by toxins, heavy metals and, most commonly, alcohol must be considered. Intracerebral causes include encephalitis, tumour and epilepsy. In the elderly, delirium often occurs following anaesthesia and surgery. Psychoactive drugs such as benzodiazepines, tricyclic antidepressants, anticonvulsants and antiparkinsonian drugs cause delirium. So do beta-blockers and digoxin.

1.21 What is the clinical course of delirium?

Delirium is of relatively rapid onset over the course of several days. In most cases it subsides once the cause has been identified and treated. However, it can persist and it might be necessary to seek further, previously unidentified, causative factors. The mortality of patients with delirium in hospital is higher than those without, and length of stay in hospital is greater.

1.22 What is the difference between delirium and dementia?

Delirium usually responds to appropriate medical treatment of the underlying cause. But if this cause is not identified (because the patient is assumed to be dementing) the consequences can be fatal. Hence it is vital to distinguish delirium from dementia and to screen for possible physical disorders in patients presenting with unexplained cognitive impairment:

■ Dementia usually has a slow, insidious course; delirium has a rapid onset.
■ In delirium, cognitive impairment and alertness fluctuate markedly, with confusion typically being worse at night. Patients with dementia usually have no loss of alertness.
■ Hallucinations and delusions are more florid in delirium, and the emotional changes are more prominent.

Patients with dementia are at an increased risk of developing delirium and, in older people, the two conditions often coexist. Dementia frequently becomes apparent for the first time after an episode of delirium has apparently failed to resolve completely, leaving a residual cognitive deficit.

1.23 How can misdiagnosis be avoided?

The keys to differentiating delirium and dementia are as follows:

■ obtain accurate information about the onset and course of symptoms from someone who knows the patient well
■ be alert to the possibility of (possibly trivial) physical illness causing dramatic cognitive changes
■ be willing and able to undertake the physical examination and clinical investigations necessary to determine causative pathology.

1.24 What is pseudodementia?

Some patients with severe depression present with loss of motivation, slowness of thought or actions, and poor concentration. They can appear to have great difficulty in attending to what one says to them and have problems recalling information. Other depressed patients might show such severe psychomotor retardation that communication, let alone objective assessment, is difficult. Such patients might initially be thought to be suffering from dementia but normally respond to conventional antidepressant therapy and their apparent cognitive deficit usually improves.

Depression in older patients can present as behavioural disturbance or functional impairment, which, again, can be mistaken for dementia. Such 'symptoms' can include increased dependence on family or neighbours, aggression or irritability, social withdrawal or incontinence.

1.25 Do patients with depression experience lasting memory problems?

A proportion of depressed older patients show significant cognitive abnormalities on neuropsychological testing. But resolution of their depression does not always result in the full resolution of their cognitive dysfunction. Such patients are more likely to have abnormal brain CT scans (typically ventricular enlargement) and the risk of them developing dementia is higher than the general population. Also, a small proportion of patients with chronic depression who have undergone numerous courses of electroconvulsive therapy (ECT) have reported lasting memory impairment.

1.26 Which other psychiatric disorders might be mistaken for dementia?

Several other psychiatric disorders can mimic dementia. These include hypomania and schizophrenia, particularly if the patient is disorganized, agitated, incoherent or showing signs of neglect. Less commonly, patients can demonstrate apparent amnesia or other cognitive impairment as the result of a so-called hysterical or somatoform disorder (e.g. Ganser syndrome).

1.27 How can depression be distinguished from early dementia?

As indicated above, dementia in its early stages can mimic depression. Presenting features of dementia often include impaired motivation and a restriction of the patient's usual range of interests. However, the onset of dementia is typically a slow and insidious one, whereas depression has a quicker onset and precipitating factors such as a significant life event can often be identified (*Table 1.2*).

Patients with dementia do not typically complain of low mood, suicidal thoughts or feelings of worthlessness unless they are also depressed. Appetite is usually normal in the early stages of dementia. The sleep pattern

Table 1.2 Features distinguishing depression with memory problems from dementia

	Depression	Dementia
History	Onset and decline often rapid with identifiable trigger factor or life event	Vague, insidious onset. Often no obvious precipitant. Symptoms progress slowly
	Symptoms become obvious early on	Symptoms might go unnoticed for years
Symptoms	Subjective complaints of memory loss	Patients often unaware or attempt to hide problems
	Symptoms often worse in the morning	Confusion often worse in evening
Mental state	Patients distressed/unhappy. Variability in cognitive performance. 'Don't know' answers	Mood might be labile. Cognitive performance consistent. Questions answered incorrectly but patients attempt them

in depression is characteristic, with interrupted sleep and early waking. Insomnia and nocturnal wandering occurs in dementia, but usually at a later stage.

It is vital that information is also sought from someone who has witnessed these changes, heard statements suggesting depression or suicidality statements or can confirm any precipitating factors.

Depressed patients are more likely to complain of memory problems than patients with dementia. On assessing cognitive function, patients with dementia usually try to answer the questions but might confabulate when doing so. Incorrect responses are often accompanied by quite plausible attempts to rationalize, although some patients become quite irritable or distressed ('catastrophic reaction'). Depressed patients are more likely not to attempt an answer and to respond by saying 'I don't know'. They are less likely to show defects of higher cortical functions such as dysphasia or dyspraxia.

Lastly, if there is still doubt, a trial of antidepressant therapy, e.g. an SSRI, should be considered. It is important to remember that patients with dementia can also become depressed. This should be treated in the usual way.

1.28 What is the connection between dementia and learning disability?

Standards of care for patients with learning disability have greatly improved and more are surviving into middle or late adulthood. As a consequence, more will develop dementia. There is a particular association between Down's syndrome and Alzheimer's disease (*see Q 10.24*). However, in general the onset of dementia is easily missed in patients with a learning disability, particularly those with severe language or functional impairment. Patients typically present with a decline in functional ability for no obvious reason. Standard tests of cognitive function are unlikely to be useful.

PATIENT QUESTIONS

1.29   Is dementia the same as ageing?

Although dementia gets very common in the 'older old age' group, i.e. over 80 years of age, it is not an inevitable consequence of ageing. Many of the common, chronic physical disorders found in older people, such as high blood pressure, diabetes and atherosclerosis do increase the chances of developing dementia. On the other hand, many of the common pathological 'markers' of dementia, e.g. signs of cerebral ischaemia and senile plaques (*see Q 10.21*) are a frequent finding at postmortem in patients who have had no memory problems before their death.

The mild forgetfulness that becomes much more common as people grow older is not dementia (*see Qs 1.7 and 1.8*).

1.30   I am worried that my memory is getting worse, should I see my GP?

Yes. Whatever the reason for your memory problem it makes sense to get it checked as soon as possible because treatment might well be available. It is possible that your forgetfulness or lack of concentration is a symptom of one of a range of medical or psychological conditions that your GP can diagnose, treat or refer on for specialist advice. Importantly, your GP might well be able to reassure you that there is nothing to be concerned about.

1.31   What should I expect my GP to do?

Your GP should ask you what you have noticed, how long it has been going on, how it started, whether it is getting worse and how your problems affect your daily life. It might also be helpful for your GP to talk to a relative or friend who knows you well. You will have to do a brief memory test and have a full physical examination. Your GP will then order blood tests and perhaps a urine test and chest X-ray. Other tests will depend on the findings from these examinations and your medical history. Your GP will then advise on treatment, request a specialist opinion or refer you on to other agencies such as social services for additional help.

1.32 What forms of dementia run in families?

A large number of forms of dementia run in families, but most of these are very rare. The usual forms of inheritance are autosomal dominant, in which up to 50% of children of an affected parent will develop the disease, and autosomal recessive, in which 25% of children will develop a dementia if both parents carry the disease gene.

The common degenerative dementias such as Alzheimer's disease, frontotemporal dementia (FTD) and dementia with Lewy bodies all have familial forms. These familial forms are unusual:

■ familial forms of frontotemporal dementia probably account for about 25% of all cases
■ familial forms of Alzheimer's disease account for about 10% of all cases of Alzheimer's disease
■ familial forms of dementia with Lewy bodies account for fewer than 10% of cases.

A number of dementias only occur in genetic forms. The most common autosomal dominant dementia is Huntington's disease (*see* Q 1.33). Other genetic diseases include CADASIL and mitochondrial disease.

The recessive forms of dementia include Wilson's disease and many glycogen and lipid storage diseases.

1.33 When will cures for genetic dementias be available?

The discovery of the genetic causes of Huntington's disease, familial Alzheimer's and one form of frontotemporal dementia have not yet led to dramatic new treatments for these diseases. The genes for these diseases were discovered only in the last 10 years and it is still too early to expect new treatments.

One obvious new method of treatment would be to manufacture good copies of the gene to replace mutant genes in affected individuals. The problem so far with this approach is the difficulty of delivering the new gene to brain cells without damaging them.

As far as new drugs are concerned, numerous safety checks are needed and the progress from initial breakthrough to marketed drug is a long one. Nevertheless, scientists are hopeful of finding a cure through drugs and other approaches. A vaccine that slows the development of the pathological features of Alzheimer's disease in transgenic mice has been developed and was recently tested (unsuccessfully) in humans.

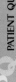

The assessment of dementia

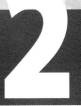

ASSESSING DEMENTIA

2.1 How is dementia assessed?

A comprehensive assessment of dementia goes beyond determining the extent of the patient's memory loss. First, dementia must be confirmed and other conditions that can mimic it ruled out. This will require a full physical and neurological examination, blood tests and possibly other investigations. It also involves interviewing both patient and, wherever possible, an informant who has witnessed the development of the patient's symptoms first hand. A full history and a mental state examination should also identify other associated psychopathology, such as mood disorder or hallucinations, and 'problem behaviours'. Cognitive assessment including the use of established rating scales will help to clarify the nature and extent of the cognitive impairment. Identification of potential risk factors and strain on carers is a vital aspect of any assessment.

Taken as a whole, this might go beyond the remit of a GP. However, a familiarity with this assessment process of assessment will help inform appropriate screening questions and tests. In turn, this will ensure that the ball starts rolling at an early stage. As well as being immensely helpful for any specialist services that subsequently become involved, it is reassuring for patients and families.

Neurologists and psychiatrists assess patients with dementia in different ways. This is partially a matter of training and interest and partially a matter of the different tasks they perform. Many neurologists see their initial (but not only) priority as making an accurate diagnosis. Many psychiatrists are more concerned with improving the quality of life of the patient more directly. Both tasks are very important in managing patients with dementia and, for this reason, many memory clinics have both a neurologist and a psychiatrist attending to optimize the management of patients.

THE ROLE OF THE GP

2.2 How should a GP approach a patient with dementia?

GPs have a vital role in the detection and continuing management of patients with dementia. The GP or another member of the primary care team is well placed to identify patients who might be developing the condition. The use of a simple rating scale such as the Mental Test Score (MTS) or Mini Mental State Examination (MMSE) can identify patients with possible dementia. This can perhaps best be done through screening programmes, e.g. by a practice nurse as part of the 'over 75' health check. The primary care service should collaborate with specialist services to ensure that such systems are in place and that staff receive sufficient training to screen patients effectively, and to act appropriately on the findings.

Despite any involvement by specialist services, the primary care team will very often be the first port of call for carers or patients seeking advice and medical support. It is important for them to be alert to changes in the lifestyle and coping abilities of patients known to them. A willingness to refer promptly to specialist psychiatric services or social services will help to avert crises in the future.

2.3 What do I need to consider when assessing dementia?

First, it is necessary to establish that a patient is suffering from dementia rather than, for example, delirium or severe depression (*see Qs 1.22–1.24*). The cause of the dementia should then be considered and, in particular, whether it is reversible or potentially life threatening.

It is useful to establish which 'domains', or areas, of cognitive function are affected, and to what extent. In addition to cognitive impairment, there might be a range of psychiatric symptoms, episodes of disturbed behaviour and problems with the activities of day-to-day living. Further aspects of the assessment include determining risk and considering management options. Exploring the effect on carers is an important part of the assessment.

This can be a lengthy process and a comprehensive assessment is beyond the scope of most GPs, if only because of time constraints. However, keeping the various elements of the assessment in mind will ensure that the major problems and risks can at least be identified, and patients referred on to the appropriate agencies.

2.4 How is an assessment carried out?

Much of the assessment is elicited through careful history taking, using information from other people as appropriate. In particular, the assessment should clearly identify those areas that are likely to represent a risk to the health, safety or wellbeing of patients and their carers or family. Information gathered during the history is supplemented by the use of rating scales, physical examination and investigations.

The conventional structured approach to taking a medical history can be used. It is necessary to identify when symptoms suggestive of dementia became apparent, what the symptoms were and how the condition has progressed since then. Any precipitating or aggravating factors should be noted, as should the history of any significant medical conditions, medication currently being taken and whether the patient uses alcohol to a significant extent. A family history of dementia should be recorded, as should details of any previous psychiatric or psychological treatment received. An assessment should include details of patients' home circumstances, support received and family members.

Appropriate examination of mental state, cognitive function and physical condition should then be performed.

2.5 Where should this assessment be carried out?

Psychiatrists usually recommend assessment in the patient's own home for a number of reasons:

- Patients are often anxious when attending a health centre or hospital department and this can interfere with accurate history taking and assessment of mental state and cognitive performance.
- An informant – a spouse or home-careworker – is more likely to be available in the patient's home to give useful collateral information.
- Even a cursory inspection of a person's surroundings can give clues as to the ability to manage. An examination of the contents of the fridge is frequently instructive. There might, for example, be little or no fresh food in the house. Direct evidence such as this often contradicts a patient's insistence that 'everything is fine'.

2.6 How do I assess cognitive impairment?

You need to consider the various cognitive domains: memory, language, praxis, recognition, visuoperceptual skills, judgement, planning, and so on. Many of these domains are interdependent and, with a few exceptions such as well-defined stroke, deficits tend to be multiple. However, the pattern of cognitive impairment taken as a whole might indicate the diagnosis or the severity of the dementia.

The level of consciousness and activity, motivation, social behaviour and mood can be determined by general observation. Drowsiness, marked apathy or severe agitation, due perhaps to delirium or advanced dementia, is likely to affect the quality of a cognitive assessment. Without these, a person might be otherwise uncooperative because of anxiety, fear, psychosis or personality change.

It is then customary to test orientation to both time (by asking the day, date, month and year) and place ('Tell me exactly where we are now').

NEUROPSYCHOLOGICAL SYMPTOMS OF DEMENTIA

2.7 What terms are used to describe the neuropsychological symptoms of dementia?

The number of different terms used by neurologists in dealing with patients with dementia is large and potentially confusing; this chapter aims to explain many of them.

The prefixes 'a' or 'dys' are often applied to words describing neurological symptoms, e.g. aphasia and dysphasia. Strictly speaking 'a' means 'absence of' – so aphasia is absence of speech – whereas 'dys' means 'problem with' – so dysphasia is a speech problem. However, both terms are now used interchangeably, with the 'a' words being used increasingly. This text will explain and use only the 'a' forms.

2.8   What is apraxia?

Apraxia is one of those terms that means different things to different people. In the strictest sense, it is a problem with the planning of a motor task (e.g. doing up a button) in the absence of a motor problem in the hand. The hand is not weak, it has normal sensation and coordination, but the patient cannot plan how to manipulate the fingers to do the task. Neurologists who see patients with dementia and other neurodegenerative diseases often use the term 'apraxia' when the *predominant* problem the patient has is planning tasks, i.e. even if there are mild problems with coordination.

The naming of the different types of apraxia is complex and is beyond this book. The two main types can be tested for by asking the patient to:

- mime actions such as combing the hair or brushing the teeth
- copy meaningless hand postures.

Apraxia can selectively affect mouth movements – actions like yawning, coughing or blowing a kiss. This is called orobuccal apraxia. It is usually associated with neurodegenerative disease and localizes to the dominant (usually left) perisylvian region.

Gait apraxia – difficulty in planning walking – is quite common. The patient has problems rising from a chair and has difficulty in starting to walk. Once started, the walking is small-stepped and unsteady. It is associated with bilateral frontal disease and is a feature of small vessel disease in particular. Virtually every GP practice or geriatric ward will have patients with a gait apraxia.

2.9   What is agnosia?

Agnosia is the inability to recognize scenes or objects despite normal visual acuity and fields. It is the result of a problem with the occipital or parietal lobes leading to an inability of the brain to process visual information, i.e. make sense of the visual input. It is subdivided into those forms when the shape of objects cannot be accurately traced (apperceptive) and forms when shapes can be traced but not named (associative).

Agnosia is usually tested by asking the patient to point to one of a series of simple line drawings, such as those in the ACE test (see Appendix 1).

2.10 What is aphasia?

Aphasia is a difficulty in speech produced by disease of the language areas of the brain. The classification of aphasia is complex but three main forms are recognized:

- expressive aphasia
- receptive aphasia
- nominal aphasia.

EXPRESSIVE APHASIA

This is an aphasia in which there are problems with the production of words. Language is understood but when patients try to speak they are unable to produce words as they would wish. It is due to disease in the dominant frontal lobe. The affected part of the lobe is called Broca's area and this form of aphasia is known as Broca's aphasia. Expressive aphasia can be tested by listening to the patient's speech, which is typically hesitant, with stumbling over words. An expressive aphasia is usually accompanied by difficulty naming real objects. The aphasia is usually more pronounced for rarely used words and the patient should be asked to name a series of objects which are of increasing difficulty such as watch, strap, buckle and winder (which can all be done with a normal watch).

RECEPTIVE APHASIA

This is an aphasia in which there are problems with the understanding of language. Patients with a receptive aphasia are not able to follow complex commands. Their speech is fluent but it does not make complete sense, the wrong word is used and sometimes new words (neologisms) are made up. Receptive aphasia is caused by disease of the dominant temporal lobe. The area involved is called Wernicke's area and this type of aphasia is sometimes called Wernicke's aphasia.

Receptive aphasias can be tested by listening to the patient's speech and then by asking the patient to do increasingly difficult tasks:

- point to the door
- point to the door after touching the wall
- touch your left ear with your right hand.

The substitution of words is also called 'paraphrasia'. There are two types of paraphrasia:

- Semantic: when the new word is related in meaning to the correct word. So the patient says 'giraffe' instead of 'zebra'.
- Phonemic: when the new word is related in sound to the correct word. So the patient says 'carrier' instead of 'caravan'.

NOMINAL APHASIA

This is a specific problem with finding the right word for an object. It is caused by problems in the dominant inferior temporal gyrus. It can be brought out by asking the patient to name real objects or drawings.

2.11 What is acalculia?

Acalculia is the inability to do sums. It is associated with disease of the dominant parietal lobe. It is tested as part of the MMSE, which asks the patient to perform serial 7s. Like many tests, this is a test not only of calculation but also of attention. It can be made simpler if the patient cannot subtract 7 from 100, by asking the patient to subtract 4 from 20, or to do even simpler sums.

2.12 What is prosopagnosia?

Prosopagnosia is the inability to recognize faces. It can be missed if the patient is assumed to have the much more common inability to remember people's names. It is normally associated with bilateral temporal lobe disease and with the non-dominant (usually right) temporal lobe atrophy rather than the dominant. It can be tested for by asking the patient to name famous people pictured in a magazine.

2.13 What is dressing apraxia?

Dressing apraxia is difficulty in putting on clothes. Shirts are put on back to front or the wrong way round or clothes are put on in the wrong order. It is associated with disease of the non-dominant parietal lobe. Putting on inappropriate clothes but putting them on correctly (fur coats in summer) is suggestive of frontal lobe disease.

2.14 How do I test memory? LO2

In day-to-day clinical testing, two forms of memory are tested: anterograde verbal memory and retrograde verbal memory.

Anterograde verbal memory is the ability to learn new information. Give the patient a fictitious name and address; read it out three times and ask the patient to repeat it back each time. Test how much the patient recollects after 5–10 minutes.

Retrograde memory is recall of events or facts learned before the onset of dementia. This includes general knowledge and personal information or autobiographical memory. In Alzheimer's disease, for example, autobiographical memory is much better for more remote facts than for recent ones. One problem is that unless you seek corroboration, you probably will not know whether the patient's recall of the past is accurate.

2.15 How do I assess language impairment?

You need to consider reading and writing skills, as well as comprehension of the written and spoken word. Listening to spontaneous speech during the interview should pick up evidence of language impairment. Nominal dysphasia can be assessed by asking the patient to name items.

2.16 How do I test for complex motor skills and recognition skills?

Tests for impairment of complex motor skills (dyspraxia) include asking a patient to mime actions, e.g. brushing teeth or playing the violin, drawing a picture or clock face, or copying a diagram. Loss of recognition (agnosias) can be explored by asking the patient to describe or verbally identify an object or to name it by feel alone.

2.17 How do I test for frontal lobe impairment?

There are many aspects to frontal lobe function, including verbal fluency, abstract thinking and motor sequencing.

Verbal fluency is tested by asking the patient to list, in 1 minute, as many words beginning with a particular letter as they can. Alternatives include naming towns or animals. Unimpaired individuals should name at least 15 with minimal repetition and error.

Abstract reasoning is affected in frontal lobe impairment. One test of this is to ask patients the meaning of a well-known proverb. They probably will not be able to grasp the analogous meaning and will instead describe it in a literal or concrete way. The similarities test involves asking patients to describe the similarity between two objects, such as an apple and a banana. Rather than assigning them to the appropriate category ('they are both fruit'), a patient with frontal impairment will again give simplistic concrete descriptions ('you can eat them') or might instead describe a difference between the two ('you eat the skin of one but not the other').

Motor sequencing is tested by demonstrating an alternating sequence of hand movements on a tabletop (fist, palm, side of hand …). Patients are asked to follow the sequence with their own hands, then to continue it after the examiner has stopped.

2.18 Which rating scales are helpful in assessing cognitive function?

Various rating scales are used to help in the assessment of cognitive impairment. The most well known are the Mental Test Score (MTS) and the Mini Mental State Examination (MMSE).

2.19 What is the Mental Test Score?

The Mental Test Score (MTS) is a short test derived from the Blessed Dementia Scale. It is a 10-item scale that is used widely as a screening test for cognitive impairment in primary care:

1. What is your age?
2. What is the time (to the nearest hour?)
3. Repeat this address after me ('... ... ...') and recall it at the end of the test.
4. What is the year?
5. What is this place called?
6. Who are these people? (nurses, doctors, etc.)
7. What is your date of birth?
8. What were the dates of the First World War?
9. What is the name of the monarch?
10. Count backwards from 20 to 1.

2.20 What does the Mental Test Score mean and what are its drawbacks?

A patient's performance on the MTS cannot provide a diagnosis but, as a rule of thumb, a score of 7 or below suggests a significant degree of cognitive impairment.

The MTS measures predominantly memory and orientation and, as such, is unlikely to pick up more subtle changes. It is also heavily dependent on the patient having a good level of language function.

2.21 What is the Mini Mental State Examination?

The MMSE assesses a wider range of cognitive function than the MTS but is still dependent on the patient's ability to comprehend and respond to verbal instruction. It tests orientation to time and place; registration and delayed recall of three words; attention and calculation; language skills, including naming, reading and writing; and visual construction (*Box 2.1*).

> **Box 2.1 MMSE sample items** (© Mini Mental LLC, Inc. by special permission of the publisher Psychological Assessment Resources, Inc.)
>
> **Orientation to time:** 'What is the date?'
> **Registration:** 'Listen carefully, I am going to say three words. You say them back after I stop. Ready? Here they are … "house" (pause), "car" (pause), "lake" (pause). Now repeat those words back to me.' [Repeat this up to five times but score only the first trial.]
> **Naming:** 'What is this?' [Point to a pencil or pen.]
> **Reading:** 'Please read this and do what it says' [Show examinee the words on the stimulus form, which are 'close your eyes'.]

2.22 How do I interpret an MMSE score?

The maximum score is 30 and the minimum score is 0. However, in practice the test is not sensitive enough to accurately rate patients with severe dementia, particularly those whose language function is severely impaired. It does not test frontal lobe function and is therefore not very helpful in assessing patients with frontotemporal dementias (FTD). Performance also depends on level of intelligence. Whereas a score below 25 strongly suggests dementia, a highly educated person might have clear evidence of dementia and still score 25 or more. Conversely, a patient who is depressed, severely anxious or dysphasic following a CVA might well score below the 'cut-off' yet not have dementia. For these reasons, the MMSE must not be used on its own as a diagnostic tool. It is, however, useful as a means of monitoring change in cognitive function over time. For example, a loss of 3 or 4 points per year is expected in untreated Alzheimer's disease. Drug trials of the acetylcholinesterase inhibitors have used changes in the MMSE as a marker of the drugs' efficacy. The MMSE is also used to measure a patient's response to the drugs in clinical practice.

2.23 What is the clock-drawing test?

Testing the ability of a patient to draw a clock has been proposed as a quick and easy method of confirming the presence of dementia. A score can be given depending on the ordering of the numbers and the positioning of the hands. Patients with dementia tend to fill in the numbers by working clockwise from the figure 12 or 1 – the spacing between the figures is usually uneven or inaccurate. Most unimpaired individuals start by writing in the 12, 3, 6 and 9 at the four quadrants before completing the rest.

Although not as sensitive or as specific as the MMSE, the clock-drawing test can be useful as a quick screening test in general practice.

2.24 What is the 'ACE'

The Addenbrooke's Cognitive Examination (ACE; *see Q 1.18 and Appendix 1*) incorporates the MMSE but provides a more detailed neuropsychological assessment including, for example, a more rigorous memory test and a test of frontal lobe function. However, it remains relatively quick and easy to perform in daily clinical practice.

2.25 Which parts of the ACE are abnormal in 'worried well' patients?

Typically, 'worried well' patients perform extremely well despite their complaints. One group of 'worried well' patients are people who consciously monitor their own performance and these patients complete the tests enthusiastically to prove to themselves they 'can do it'. In other 'worried well' patients and patients with depression there is an impression that they are not trying, when asked to recall an address their immediate reply is 'I've forgotten it' (as opposed to Alzheimer's patients, who tend to reply 'What address?') but, given a little encouragement, the whole address is usually recalled. Such patients often have more difficulty in initially registering the address than in recalling it.

2.26 Which parts of the ACE are abnormal in Alzheimer's disease?

The pattern of tests varies in the different dementias. In early Alzheimer's disease the pattern can be distinctive:

- the patient is fully orientated and scores well on attentional, naming and other tasks
- memorizing the address is done fluently but recall after 5 minutes is very poor
- failure to recall all three objects
- better verbal fluencies for the letter 'P' than for animals (normal individuals name more animals than words beginning with 'P').

In more advanced Alzheimer's disease, patients become disorientated in time and then place and visuospatial tasks become more difficult. Occasionally patients with a posterior form of atrophy do selectively badly on visuospatial tasks from the onset.

2.27 Which parts of the ACE are abnormal in dementia with Lewy bodies?

In dementia with Lewy bodies (see Chapter 13), the initial pattern is often similar to that of Alzheimer's disease but there tend to be more attentional problems. Patients' performance is more variable and they might do a test easily one session and then struggle in another session. It often appears that if they can 'engage' in the task they will do it well. Like those with Alzheimer's disease, patients with dementia with Lewy bodies usually perform poorly on assessment of visuospatial tasks.

2.28 Which parts of the ACE are abnormal in frontotemporal dementia?

The ACE (like the MMSE) was not designed to assess patients with frontotemporal dementia (FTD; see Chapter 12) and patients with early 'frontal' FTD can perform very well on the ACE, occasionally scoring virtually full marks. Verbal fluencies, especially for the letter 'P', are often affected early but this is a non-specific finding.

Patients with semantic dementia have a characteristic pattern of doing very well on orientation and attention but poorly on verbal fluencies for both letter 'P' and animals, and then scoring poorly on naming of the line drawings and on pronunciation of irregular words like 'pint' and 'soot'. Visuospatial skills are usually performed well even very late in the illness.

Patients with progressive non-fluent aphasia can perform badly because of their aphasia and fail to score points for tasks they can do but cannot give the answer to. Verbal fluencies and naming of the line drawings are performed poorly and some patients have difficulty with the repetition of words and phrases.

2.29 Which parts of the ACE are abnormal in vascular dementia?

Patients with vascular dementia (see Chapter 11) can have specific cortical problems from clinical strokes and might, for example, do poorly on visuospatial tasks if they have a hemianopia from an occipital cerebral event. Patients with small vessel disease often do the tasks slowly and are poor on verbal fluencies but might do well on more complex tasks such as recall of the learnt address – if given sufficient time.

2.30 Which patients need referral to a psychologist for neuropsychological testing?

Neuropsychological testing is a useful investigation in Alzheimer's disease and other forms of dementia. Many psychologists are skilled at recognizing Alzheimer's disease but are often less confident with the rarer forms of dementia, such as frontotemporal dementia. Psychologists can often recognize the onset of Alzheimer's disease before a neurologist and psychiatrist. Although psychometric tests can be useful at any stage of dementia, many of the tests need a fair intellectual ability to complete and therefore testing in advanced disease is often less useful.

If access to a psychologist is rationed, which it is in the UK, then patients in whom the diagnosis is in doubt – who have early dementia, mild depression or are 'worried well' – should be referred for testing. Referral to a psychologist is less important in patients with more advanced disease but can still be useful in looking for the causes of the problems or to see if there is evidence of depression plus dementia or dementia alone. Many neuropsychologists also have an important role to play in rehabilitation for patients with dementia.

2.31 Which psychometric tests suggest early Alzheimer's disease?

Some psychologists regard themselves as technicians – they give a report and let the clinician make the diagnosis. Others are clinicians as well and, having spent many years assessing patients, and 2 hours with the referred patient, can often make the diagnosis earlier and more accurately than the GP.

The tasks that patients with early Alzheimer's disease score poorly on are the delayed recall of a story. When tested immediately on recall of a story they perform well but when re-tested 30 minutes later they will have forgotten much of it. In a similar fashion, if asked to copy a complex figure (such as the Rey diagram) they perform well but if asked to copy it from memory later the figure lacks detail. Not surprisingly, they also perform poorly on more complex memory tasks.

RISK ASSESSMENT

2.32 What risks should I look out for?

A patient with dementia, especially one who lives alone, is at risk for a variety of reasons. Not all patients will be at risk, and the actual risk will depend on the form of dementia, the nature of the symptoms and support services received.
The following is a summary of the possible risks:

- Fire, electrocution, or flooding through inappropriate use of household appliances.
- Malnutrition, dehydration, food poisoning through neglect of food provision or preparation.
- Hypothermia through dressing inappropriately, compounded by an inability or refusal to heat the house properly, or by wandering out of doors.
- Falls.
- Financial exploitation (by opportunistic tradesmen, acquaintances, family members), through an inability to manage money, appraise transactions or requests etc.
- Robbery or burglary.
- Assault, emotional or sexual abuse.

ASSOCIATED PSYCHOPATHOLOGY

2.33 How do I assess other psychiatric symptoms?

These might be apparent just by casual observation. It can be obvious that patients are depressed from their appearance (lack of eye contact, tearfulness), the way they talk (inexpressive, monosyllabic) or the content of their speech (pessimistic, negative, suicidal). In other patients it might be reflected in an impairment of appetite or sleep disturbance. Similarly, patients with anxiety might outwardly display their symptoms (agitation, tremulousness) or readily volunteer how they feel. Patients with psychotic symptoms such as delusions or hallucinations might be preoccupied with their experiences and describe them in detail; alternatively their behaviour might

> **Box 2.2 Screening questions for psychiatric symptoms**
> **For depression:**
> - Do you feel low in mood most or all of the time?
> - Have you lost interest in your usual activities or pastimes?
> - Is everything a struggle at the moment?
> - What does the future hold for you?
> - Do you think life is worth living?
>
> **For anxiety:**
> - Do you feel more anxious or nervous than usual?
> - Do you get panicky for no reason?
> - Can you relax when you want to?
>
> **For psychotic symptoms:**
> - Are things happening to you that you don't understand?
> - Do unpleasant or strange thoughts come into your head, which you can't get rid of?
> - Do you think people know what you are doing and even what you are thinking?
> - Do you see or hear things that you can't explain?

suggest the existence of such symptoms (talking or muttering to themselves, shouting out for no apparent reason, staring perplexedly into space).

2.34 What questions should I ask to check for other psychiatric symptoms?

The screening questions shown in *Box 2.2* can be used to confirm the presence or otherwise of psychiatric symptoms.

2.35 What are the problems in diagnosing depression in patients with dementia?

Patients with dementia might not adequately be able to express their emotional state. Some symptoms of depression, such as impaired appetite or insomnia, are non-specific and can also occur in dementia. Other symptoms or signs characteristic of certain dementias can be mistaken for depression. These include apathy in frontotemporal dementia, emotional lability and tearfulness in vascular dementia; and slowness and lack of expression in Parkinson's disease.

2.36 What characteristics should I look for if I suspect depression?

- Sad appearance.
- Agitation.

■ Loss of interest in surroundings.
■ Diurnal variation in mood, typically worse in the morning.

ASSESSMENT OF SOCIAL FUNCTIONING

2.37 How can I assess impairment of activities of daily living (ADL)?

Activities of daily living (ADL) are of two types:

■ basic activities of self care: washing, dressing , feeding
■ instrumental activities: more complex tasks such as writing cheques, driving, shopping.

Observing patients in their home and questioning them and any carers will provide a useful measure of ADL skills. This basic information can be supplemented in specialist settings by an occupational therapy assessment of practical skills or by the use of an appropriate rating scale such as the Progressive Deterioration scale.

2.38 Which aspects of a patient's social situation should I consider?

It is important to assess a patient's social situation because it can provide clues as to the presence or otherwise of dementia. It will also influence the need for additional support and – ultimately – the decision about whether a person can continue to live at home. The two main aspects of a patient's social situation are the nature of their immediate environment and their contact with others. Aspects of the home that need to be taken into account include:

■ its general state of repair and cleanliness, including evidence of self neglect
■ safety and functioning of electrical appliances, cooker, central heating boiler, etc.
■ adequacy of lighting, heating and cooking facilities
■ evidence of an adequate diet: fresh food in the fridge, provisions in the cupboards
■ potential hazards such as uneven floors or steep stairs
■ the immediate vicinity around the house. A busy road might be a hazard but there could be amenities such as a corner shop close by.

Contact with others is important not only to provide help with daily self-care activities but also for emotional support and social stimulation. It is, therefore, useful to find out if family members visit, whether neighbours call in and any support provided through social services, such as home care and attendance at day centres or lunch clubs.

THE ROLE OF THE OLD-AGE PSYCHIATRIST

2.39 How does an old-age psychiatrist approach a patient with dementia?

Most old-age psychiatry services are community oriented. Patients referred by their GP are frequently seen in their own home for a full assessment. Wherever possible, an informant who knows the patient, such as a relative, carer or the GP, is invited to attend the interview.

Details of the nature of the individual's symptoms, and their progression over time, are recorded. Consequent problems of functioning are explored and reports of potential or actual risky behaviour are noted. In addition, a background history is taken, which includes personal and family details, medical, psychiatric and drug and alcohol history. An assessment of the patient's cognitive function is made, usually using a validated rating scale such as the MMSE (*see Qs 2.20 and 2.21*), with additional tests such as the clock-drawing test (*see Q 2.22*) and tests of abstract thinking and verbal fluency. A mental state examination is also conducted to determine if there is any mood disturbance, anxiety or psychosis (such as delusions or hallucinations; *see Chapter 3*).

A preliminary diagnosis is made on the basis of this assessment. Any further investigations are identified, as are the patient's needs for treatment and social care. The needs of a spouse or other carer are also taken into account.

The old-age psychiatrist is then responsible for communicating these findings to the GP and for liaising with other health or social agencies to provide appropriate ongoing care.

THE ROLE OF THE NEUROLOGIST

2.40 How does a neurologist assess a patient with dementia?

This, of course, depends on the neurologist, the time available to see the patient and the resources available. The first part of the assessment is the referral letter from the GP (*see Q 2.41*). The letter should include the 'brief', i.e. what the referring GP expects from the neurologist.

The next part of the assessment is the interview with the patient. Ideally, the neurologist should conduct the interview in three stages, starting with the patient alone, then with the patient and spouse and then with the spouse alone. The last is best achieved without embarrassment by speaking to the spouse as the patient prepares for the physical examination in a different room. Questionnaires for spouses and patients are often useful to cover parts of the history.

The patient should be examined cognitively and physically. Although the ACE (see Appendix 1) includes the items of the MMSE, it does not cover all cognitive domains and apraxia should be tested for by asking the patient to copy meaningless hand postures and mime brushing their teeth with a toothbrush; frontal lobe function can be assessed by asking for some cognitive estimates and for the meanings of common proverbs (*see Q 2.17*).

Following the examination, if the patient has severe cognitive problems it might be a good idea to speak first with the spouse alone (as the patient dresses), otherwise speak to both together.

The lack of a partner is a major handicap to the assessment. The combination of a patient coming alone and a GP letter that fails to give sufficient background can make it very difficult to diagnose even patients with severe cognitive problems.

2.41 What should be included in a referral letter to a neurologist?

A good referral letter does three things:

- ■ it acts as a record of the patient's history and examination at a particular time
- ■ it asks for an appointment (and may ask for an early or urgent appointment)
- ■ it instructs the specialist.

A good letter is usually about ½ page long. The history should make clear who is the prime mover in asking for the referral – the patient, the spouse or the GP. The level of previous functioning of the patient, the major complaint and an anecdote illustrating the problem are useful. Other parts of the history, such as past medical history and family history, should be included if relevant. The patient's medication should be listed. Positive, relevant examination findings are rare but important. Long lists of normal examination findings are unhelpful.

Some GPs are shy of telling hospital doctors what to do but it is nearly always helpful if they do so. GPs should also comment on how they think the patient has changed. A GP who has known the patient well for 15 years has a much clearer perspective on a patient than a specialist who sees the patient once for 30 minutes. Copies of letters of previous relevant assessment are usually more helpful than a brief précis.

Figure 2.1 is an example of a good referral letter.

EXAMINING PATIENTS WITH DEMENTIA

2.42 How important is a general medical examination in patients with dementia?

The importance of the general medical examination is related to the length of the history. Patients with a subacute encephalopathy (who have a history of cognitive problems lasting days to weeks) will often have physical signs

The surgery
The street
The town
The county
The postcode

The date

Dear Dr Smith

Mr Harold Weasenham

I would be grateful if you would send an early appointment to see Harold Weasenham, a 58-year-old university lecturer. His wife and I are very concerned about his behaviour; he is not. For the last 9 months he has become apathetic and reclusive. I wondered if he was depressed and asked our psychiatrist, Dr Jones, to see him; I enclose his letter. In the last month Harold has started stealing sweets from the village shop. I have known him for 15 years and this is completely out of character. I agree with Dr Jones that Harold seems to be developing an organic dementia.

Harold has been hypertensive for 5 years and is on bendrofluazide 2.5 mg but no other medication. His father died of Alzheimer's disease at the age of 63 years. I could find no abnormal neurological signs. He did well on answering simple questions of orientation.

He needs to be seen soon, to decide whether he can continue in his current post or should seek early retirement on medical grounds.

Yours sincerely,

Susan Rogers, GP

▲

Fig. 2.1 A good referral letter.

on examination relevant to their cognitive problems; patients with a longer history usually have a normal general examination. The typical causes of an encephalopathy include liver and renal failure, hypoxia from respiratory failure and other metabolic disturbances such as diabetic ketoacidosis. The number of possible physical signs pointing to these diagnoses is large but some are very typical – asterixis (liver flap) is seen in most patients presenting with hepatic encephalopathy (it is also seen in respiratory failure and other conditions).

In patients with a dementia it is important to look for evidence of vascular disease by:

■ measuring the blood pressure
■ examining the blood vessels of the retina and the optic nerve head
■ examining the peripheral pulses.

It is important to check for signs of other medical conditions, such as hypothyroidism, that might be contributing to the patient's problems.

The medical examination in the majority of patients with dementia does not help the diagnosis but the number of potentially relevant physical signs is large.

2.43 What do I need to look for in a neurological examination in a patient with dementia?

The neurological examination still carries a mystique. The number of signs that might be present in a patient with dementia is very large but, in practice, only a few of them are likely to alter the management of the patient. Most doctors will never see a patient with dementia through vitamin B_{12} deficiency or due to a leukodystrophy.

Box 2.3 highlights those parts of the examination that are occasionally abnormal and, when abnormal, alter the management of the patient.

VISUAL FIELDS

Visual fields are important. A typical finding is a right upper quadrantinopia in a patient with language disturbance; this suggests a problem in the left temporal lobe. In a patient with acute onset of problems this suggests a stroke; in a patient with progressive problems a tumour.

Box 2.3 The most informative parts of the neurological examination in patients with dementia
■ General appearance and facial expression
■ Visual fields
■ Fundoscopy
■ Movement and gait

Patients who have difficulty in localizing objects in space bilaterally (e.g. who, when asked to grab a wriggling finger, fail to do so) usually have degenerative disease of the parieto-occipital lobes (usually due to Alzheimer's disease or dementia with Lewy bodies).

FUNDOSCOPY

Examination of the optic disc will occasionally reveal papilloedema, suggesting that the patient has raised intracranial pressure; in a patient with dementia this usually means a tumour.

Features of Parkinson's disease are often present in patients with degenerative dementia. Parkinson's disease is best diagnosed as the patient walks into the room from the staring face, reduced arm swing and shuffling gait. Parkinsonism is a prominent feature of dementia with Lewy bodies but is also seen in patients with Alzheimer's disease and frontotemporal dementia.

GAIT

The gait of the patient is the final important part of the neurological assessment. There are a number of different gaits, which provide important clues to the underlying diagnosis:

- A small-stepped, unsteady gait and difficulty in getting up from the chair and initiating movements is typical of small-vessel disease. This gait is sometimes called *marché a petit pas* or an apraxic gait.
- A stooped gait with reduced arm swing and a staring face and a tendency to turn *en bloc* is typical of Parkinson's disease.
- A subtle hemiplegic gait suggests a stroke or tumour, often most noticeable as the patient walks.
- A wide-based, stiff-legged gait is typical of multiple sclerosis.

There are other neurological gaits which might be relevant in occasional patients.

2.44 What are the 'release reflexes'?

The presence of release reflexes suggests organic disease but their value in discriminating organic dementia from non-organic cognitive problems is overstated in many books.

Release reflexes are also called 'primitive reflexes' and 'frontal release signs'. They are reflexes that are present in the neonatal child and which reappear in degenerative dementias. They do not localize the disease to the frontal lobes. Although their presence is an indicator of organic brain disease, some can be seen in normal individuals. There are several (*Fig. 2.2*), of which the most important are:

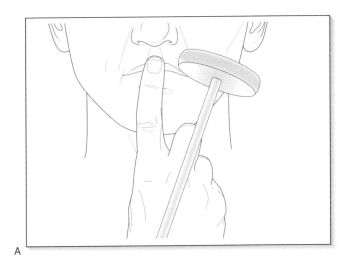

A

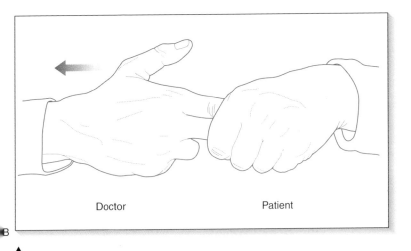

Doctor   Patient

B

Fig. 2.2 Four release reflexes. A. Pout: the lips are tapped lightly with a tendon hammer, as shown. In a positive response they pucker. B. Grasp: the two fingers are drawn across the patient's palm. The patient grasps the fingers involuntarily. C. Palmomental: the palm is scratched with an orange stick and the contralateral chin puckers. D. Visual rooting: the patient's head turns and the mouth opens in response to the approach of an object.

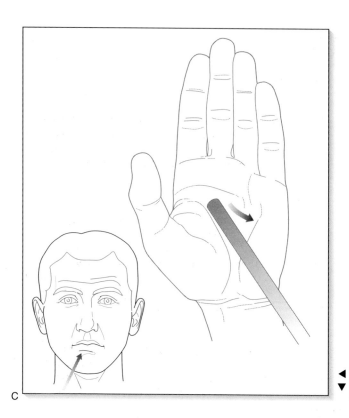

C

Fig. 2.2
(cont'd)

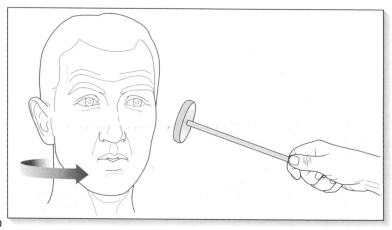

D

■ pout reflex
■ rooting reflex
■ grasp reflex
■ palmomental reflex.

POUT REFLEX

The pout reflex is elicited when the examiner places a finger vertically (and lightly) on the patient's lips. The examiner's finger is then lightly tapped with a tendon hammer. If the lips pucker the reflex is present. The pout reflex is not a good discriminating, and is seen in normal individuals with increasing age and not a true release reflex.

ROOTING REFLEX

To elicit the rooting reflex one cheek is gently tickled with an orange stick or similar object. In a positive test the patient turns the head towards the stimulus in the way that a baby turns towards a breast or bottle. In patients with advanced disease, the head and mouth turn towards a visually presented stimulus. The rooting reflex might be accompanied by opening of the mouth. The presence of a clear visual rooting reflex is an indicator of an organic dementia. It is usually seen in advanced disease.

GRASP REFLEX

This is elicited by stroking across the patient's palm, towards the thumb. A positive response occurs when the patient closes the hand into a fist and grasps the examiner's fingers. The response is involuntary and needs to be distinguished from a voluntary response by asking the patient to try to suppress the clenching.

Grasp reflexes are seen in patients with organic disease. A unilateral response is occasionally present in focal contralateral frontal lobe disease and is an indication for CT/MRI scanning.

PALMOMENTAL REFLEX

This is produced by scratching the patient's palm with a blunt stick such as an orange stick. When the reflex is present the contralateral chin puckers. It is a late sign of organic brain disease.

2.45 What investigations should a GP organize in a patient with suspected dementia?

Physical investigations are necessary in suspected dementia for three reasons. First, to exclude other physical conditions that might mimic dementia or cause so-called 'reversible dementia'. These are many and varied but those that can be identified through simple blood screening are:

■ vitamin B_{12} deficiency
■ hypothyroidism
■ heavy alcohol consumption (gamma GT and MCV)
■ hypercalcaemia.

Second, to help confirm or rule out delirium. Blood screening will help exclude causes such as dehydration (urea and creatinine), hyponatraemia (serum sodium), anaemia and infection (white cell count). A general physical examination should exclude obvious foci of infection, such as a respiratory tract infection; and constipation. Further investigations such as a midstream urine (MSU) culture and chest X-ray might then be indicated.

Third, it is necessary to check for any physical sequelae of dementia, for example the effects of poor nutrition (protein deficiency) or dehydration.

In summary, a GP is normally asked to organize a 'dementia screen', which, as well as a full physical examination, usually comprises:

■ full blood count (FBC)
■ erythrocyte sedimentation rate (ESR)
■ renal function tests – urea and electrolytes (U&E), creatinine
■ liver function tests (LFT) – bilirubin, albumin and liver enzymes including gamma glutamyl transferase
■ thyroid function tests (TFT)
■ serum glucose and calcium
■ vitamin B_{12} and folate
■ MSU, ECG and chest X-ray, if clinically indicated.

IMAGING

2.46 What types of scan are used to assess a patient with dementia?

There are two main types of brain scan:

■ structural scans, e.g. MRI and CT: show the topography of the brain
■ functional scans, e.g. SPECT and PET: measure the function of the brain.

Structural scans are much more widely used in clinical practice than functional scans (*see Qs 2.47 and 2.48*).

Two types of structural brain scan are commonly used in the assessment of patients with dementia: a magnetic resonance imaging (MRI) scan or a computerized tomographic (CT) scan. In general, a MRI scan is preferable – it gives higher quality images and more detail of the structure of the brain. For example, an MRI scan can show the degree of atrophy in different lobes of the brain and is very sensitive to changes in the white matter due to vascular disease. Therefore, patients with dementia should generally have an

MRI scan. However, there are a number of good reasons why a physician might choose to order a CT scan instead:

■ having an MRI scan can be very unpleasant, especially if the patient is claustrophobic
■ the patient needs to be able to stay very still for about 15 minutes to have a routine MRI scan
■ patients with metal implants, such as pacemakers, cannot have MRI scans
■ CT scans are much more readily available in many parts of the country and can often be arranged more quickly than MRI scans.

2.47 Is there a role for SPECT scanning in dementia?

Single photon emission computed tomography (SPECT) scans are widely available and are the only functional scan used in routine clinical practice; most departments of nuclear medicine can perform one. However, their role is limited. Although SPECT is a sensitive way to diagnose cerebral tumours and other problems, structural scans such as CT and MRI fulfil this role far better. The main roles of SPECT are to:

■ Show reduced blood flow secondary to dementia. These changes can be visualized earlier by SPECT than by the structural scans. This is particularly useful in the identification of early frontal lobe dementias when a patient has a questionable behavioural or personality change. A SPECT scan showing reduced blood flow in the frontal lobes suggests the problems reflect an organic dementia.
■ Distinguish Alzheimer's disease from frontotemporal dementia.

SPECT scan results should be interpreted cautiously if they are out of keeping with other assessments. They are a guide to the diagnosis and not a replacement for structural imaging.

2.48 Are PET scans more reliable than SPECT?

Yes, positron emission tomography (PET) scans are the most sensitive guide in the early diagnosis of dementia and reveal changes earlier than structural scans such as MRI. In Alzheimer's disease, a bilateral parieto-occipital pattern of hypometabolism or reduced blood flow is seen; in FTD frontal hypometabolism is seen. PET is sensitive enough to show differences between the two sides of the brain and within lobes. Unfortunately, a cyclotron – a machine capable of producing positrons (which decay very rapidly) is required, and these are extremely expensive. PET scanning has other drawbacks, although these can be overcome – if metabolism is to be measured then arterial blood samples are needed and a small amount of radioactivity is injected.

The need for a cyclotron means that most dementia specialists have learnt to diagnose dementias without the benefit of PET scans and, in the UK, they are mainly a research tool.

2.49 Is there a role for an EEG in the diagnosis of dementia?

Prior to the development of structural imaging in the form of CT scans, the electroencephalogram (EEG) was often used as a screen for dementia as opposed to non-organic disease, to detect brain tumours and to distinguish Alzheimer's disease from frontal dementias. These days, more modern and sensitive techniques are available. However, an EEG can still be a useful test:

■ slowing of the dominant rhythm is an indicator of an organic dementia
■ patients with Creutzfeldt–Jakob disease might have a florid (but not specific) abnormality of periodic triphasic complexes
■ it is normal in the early stages of FTD and can be a pointer towards FTD rather than Alzheimer's disease.

2.50 Which patients with dementia require a lumbar puncture?

Although some patients with dementia have a lumbar puncture as part of their investigations, it is rare for the results of the cerebrospinal fluid analysis to change the management of the patient. The test is usually done as part of the 'let's leave no stone unturned' approach to medicine in patients who are young, have abnormal MRI scans, have a rapidly progressive history or other concerning features.

 PATIENT QUESTIONS

2.51 What is a SPECT scan?

SPECT stands for single photon emission computed tomography. A SPECT scan is a scan in which a small amount of radioactivity is used to give a picture of the brain. It is a functional scan – this means that the picture is produced by activity of the brain (usually based on the blood flow to the brain) rather than the actual structure.

2.52 If my wife has had a CT scan for dementia does she need an MRI scan as well?

Virtually all treatable conditions will show up on a CT scan of the head in a patient with established dementia. So the vast majority of patients who have had a CT head scan do not require a later MRI head scan. However, it might be suggested if doubt remains about the diagnosis or if the doctors involved have a research interest in the dementias.

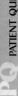

2.53 Do patients with dementia develop swallowing problems?

Swallowing problems are a common feature of Alzheimer's disease and other forms of dementia. The difficulties can be caused by a number of factors, including difficulty planning the complex action of swallowing or weakness in the swallowing muscles. Sometimes there is a simple cause, such as false teeth that no longer fit but the patient is unable to say this. Swallowing problems are seen in all forms of dementia but if they are troublesome early in the illness then conditions such as progressive supranuclear palsy and motor neuron disease dementia need to be considered.

2.54 How are swallowing problems treated in patients with dementia?

Very often, the treatment of swallowing problems is a matter of patience and common sense – looking for simple problems such as poor eating posture and poorly fitting false teeth. Semisolid foods are generally easier to swallow than solid ones. Advice from a speech therapist is often useful. Medical intervention is sometimes needed and a small operation to insert a feeding tube into the stomach – a percutaneous gastrostomy or PEG – can significantly improve the quality of life in some patients.

2.55 Is weight change a feature of dementia?

Yes. Both weight loss and weight gain can be problems in dementia.

Weight loss occurs in many patients, usually in the later stages of dementia. It is seen in Alzheimer's disease, vascular dementia and the other common dementias. It seems to be a combination of reduced appetite and increased difficulty in eating/swallowing.

Weight loss is best treated with regular small meals, although the occasional patient requires feeding with a percutaneous gastrostomy.

Weight gain is a feature of frontotemporal dementia and is due to overeating. It can be a real problem if access to food is unrestricted. Some patients will eat everything put in front of them but will not seek-out food, some will eat only sweet foods. Others will seek-out and eat any form of food. Weight gain can be treated by restricting access to food or the overeating can be treated successfully sometimes with some of the newer antidepressants – selective serotonin reuptake inhibitors (SSRIs), although this is not a licensed indication.

Psychiatric symptoms and behavioural changes in dementia

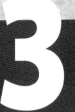

3.1 What kind of psychological or behavioural changes are seen in dementia?

A wide range of psychiatric and emotional conditions frequently occurs in patients with dementia. Mood changes, particularly lability of mood and depression, are common. Psychotic symptoms include hallucinations in various modalities – visual, auditory, somatic – and delusional beliefs. Such symptoms can indicate specific types of dementia, the onset of delirium or herald an overall decline in the patient's condition. These are often accompanied by degrees of behavioural disturbance such as agitation, wandering or sleep disruption. Psychiatric symptoms and behavioural changes contribute greatly to carer burden and increase the likelihood of the patient being unable to manage, or be managed, safely in the community. Questions relating to the drug treatment of these symptoms can be found in Chapter 6.

DISORDERS OF MOOD IN DEMENTIA

3.2 What mood changes occur in dementia?

Patients with dementia demonstrate mood changes of various forms. Patients with all types of dementia can experience anxiety, irritability or low mood during the course of their illness. Dementia with Parkinson's disease is closely linked to depression and anxiety. The frontal lobe dementias are characterized by changes in personality, which often involves anger and hostility.

3.3 What is 'emotional lability'?

Patients with emotional lability demonstrate frequent and unpredictable changes in emotion, with brief periods of tearfulness, elation, or irritability occurring with little or no provocation. Vascular dementia, in particular, is associated with emotional lability. The patient might deny that they experience the distress or other emotional extreme that they appear to express.

3.4 How can mood change be identified in a severely demented patient?

Assessment of mood changes in dementia can be difficult if there is loss of language function. Observed behaviour that might indicate that an uncommunicative patient with dementia is depressed include:

■ agitation
■ irritability
■ slowness of speech or movement

■ onset of appetite or sleep disturbance
■ a lack of interest in surroundings or previously enjoyed activity.

Patients with depression or anxiety as well as dementia are likely to perform less well in activities of daily living (ADL), thus increasing the need for support, or residential care.

3.5 How common is depression in dementia?

One or more symptoms of depression occur in up to 50% of patients with dementia. Studies indicate that the prevalence of actual depressive disorder is around 20%.

3.6 Why do patients with dementia get depressed?

In the early stages of dementia, when insight is retained, depression can be part of the individual's adjustment reaction to the implications of the diagnosis. Not all patients with dementia become depressed. The patient's psychological resources and coping skills, and support network will influence the risk of depression. There is no evidence that withholding the diagnosis lessens this risk; indeed knowing there is 'something wrong, but I don't know what' can be more, not less, distressing.

Depression in the later stages of the dementia is more likely to be caused by the effects of the cerebral degeneration itself.

3.7 Which factors increase the risk of depression in patients with dementia?

Patients with dementia who have a past history or a positive family history of depressive disorder are more likely themselves to develop depression. Other risk factors – as with patients without dementia – include social isolation, chronic and painful physical illness, and bereavement.

3.8 Does the prevalence of depression differ according to the type of dementia?

Most studies have concluded that vascular dementia and dementia with Lewy bodies are more commonly associated with depression than is Alzheimer's disease. Frontotemporal dementia appears less likely to cause depression.

3.9 Do patients with dementia attempt suicide?

Yes. But there is little information about the incidence of suicide attempts in patients with dementia compared with other elderly populations. A suicide attempt might occur in the context of a coexisting depressive episode. It might also be a considered act, taken following a lucid appraisal of the implications of the dementia for that individual. Dementia in Huntington's disease is most commonly associated with suicide.

3.10 Why do patients with dementia get anxious?

Anxiety is common. Patients with dementia who have sufficient insight might be appropriately anxious over their condition and what their future will hold. Anxiety might also be a reaction to changes in routine or other situations that the patient cannot fully understand. Fear or perplexity is often the result of hallucinations or delusions.

3.11 What are the implications of anxiety in a patient with dementia?

Decline in functional ability and consequent loss of confidence increases anxiety. This causes further decline in ability, setting up a vicious cycle of increasing dependency on a spouse or other carer. Increased anxiety then supervenes if that carer is not present. This often results in a sufferer not wanting to be left alone – or even out of sight – even for very short periods of time. This, of course, gets very wearing for even the most devoted carer.

3.12 What is the catastrophic reaction?

> The catastrophic reaction is an extreme emotional reaction to difficulty in accomplishing an activity. It may be seen during an assessment of cognitive function or whilst attempting ordinary household tasks. The reaction takes the form of sudden screaming; angry or violent outbursts, such as striking out. It is more likely to occur when the patient is severely cognitively impaired and where there is co-existing delirium, psychotic symptoms or mood changes. People caring for patients with dementia – at home or in residential care – need to be aware that this can occur; often with no warning.

PSYCHOSIS IN DEMENTIA

3.13 Which psychotic symptoms occur in dementia?

The two main psychotic symptoms are hallucinations and delusions. Hallucinations are defined as 'perceptions occurring in the absence of a stimulus'. They are typically vivid and lifelike, occurring in external space. These perceptions can be in any sensory modality but visual and auditory hallucinations are most common.

Delusions are abnormal beliefs that are held with a firm conviction in the absence of confirmatory evidence. The beliefs are not in keeping with social, cultural or religious norms.

3.14 How common are hallucinations in dementia?

Hallucinations occur in up to 20–30% of patients with Alzheimer's disease. They are much more prevalent in patients with dementia with Lewy bodies (70–80%) and also occur frequently in patients with vascular dementia.

Visual hallucinations are the most common form in all types of dementia, followed by auditory hallucinations.

3.15 What form do the hallucinations take?

Visual hallucinations often take the form of 'small people', or children, in the home. They are typically vivid. Illusions, where a viewed object is mistaken for something else are commonly experienced during evening or night when the light is dim. So-called extracampine visual hallucinations are more complex. Here, patients describe seeing themselves or their home and its contents from an unusual angle, e.g. as if they were flying above, or from beyond the normal field of view.

Auditory hallucinations take various forms but are not usually as elaborate as in psychotic conditions such as schizophrenia. In dementia, auditory hallucinations can be simple conversations, voices speaking, or music.

Although hallucinations can be distressing or unnerving, they can also be a source of comfort or entertainment to a person living alone.

3.16 What is Charles Bonnet syndrome?

Charles Bonnet syndrome is the combination of vivid visual hallucinations that occurs in elderly patients in clear consciousness and with no apparent cognitive impairment. The patient invariably has some loss of visual acuity. It occurs most commonly where the patient is socially isolated. The hallucinations are vivid but the patient is usually able to accept that they are the result of their 'eyes playing tricks'.

3.17 What forms of delusions occur in dementia?

Delusions of various kinds are common in dementia. Examples include the belief that carers or nursing staff are poisoning food, that a spouse is having an affair with the home help or that intruders are breaking in and rearranging furniture. Patients might incorporate what they have seen on television into their own reality. One patient had watched the news on television and the next day described a recent holiday to Yemen during which she had been caught up in a terrorist attack. Delusional misidentification occurs where a patient insists that a stranger has replaced a spouse or other familiar figure (Capgras' syndrome). The patient usually acknowledges that the 'imposter' looks exactly the same as the spouse.

It should not be automatically assumed that firmly held beliefs are delusional. Complaints such as 'they are all trying to get me out of my home' or 'my daughter has been stealing my jewellery' might turn out to be true.

3.18 What is the 'mirror sign'?

This is a form of delusional misidentification in which patients believe that their own reflected image in a mirror is another person. They might attempt a conversation with this image, or report an 'intruder' in their home.

3.19 What causes the psychotic symptoms of dementia?

Various brain regions, including the temporal, parietal and frontal lobes, have all been implicated in the development of delusional beliefs in dementia. However, delusions can also be understood as a faulty attempt by individuals to make sense of a situation that they cannot fully grasp or that has become unfamiliar. For example, patients with moderate or severe dementia who are having difficulty managing at home but refusing home care might well live in tatty or squalid surroundings. They might attribute the untidiness to intruders entering their home and disturbing their belongings. The loss of an item of value through forgetfulness could lead to the belief that the cleaner has stolen it. The Police are frequently called in these circumstances.

3.20 Which types of dementia are associated with psychosis?

Patients with all types of dementia can experience psychotic symptoms. However, both vascular dementia and, in particular, dementia with Lewy bodies are characterized by visual hallucinations, and delusional beliefs are very commonly seen. Some forms of vascular dementia, notably Binswanger's disease, can present with psychotic conditions such as delusional disorders, even before the onset of cognitive impairment.

3.21 What are the other risk factors for psychosis in dementia?

Coexisting sensory impairment such as hearing loss or impairment of visual acuity (cataracts, macular degeneration) increase the risk of hallucinations. This risk is compounded by social isolation. The effects of television have already been mentioned. Although we are not aware of any studies looking at this scientifically, it seems likely that if television is the sole source of cerebral stimulation or social interaction then a weakened grip on reality is inevitable.

3.22 What are the other causes of psychosis in dementia?

Although the onset of delusions or hallucinations might just be a 'stage' of the dementing illness, two other possibilities need to be considered. First, delirium secondary to, for example, infection or prescribed drugs can cause vivid visual or auditory hallucinations; as can delusional beliefs, which are frequently distressing but might well not be described clearly by the patient. Second, but less commonly, severe depression with psychotic symptoms is associated with second-person auditory hallucinations (i.e. voices talking to the patient), the content of which might be obscene, derogatory or threatening. Depression is also associated with delusions of persecution, hypochondriasis (abnormal beliefs about one's state of health or physical symptoms) or nihilism – extremely negative abnormal beliefs, for example regarding the loss or destruction of one's money, home, belongings and even body.

3.23 Do psychotic symptoms have a prognostic significance?

Patients with hallucinations are more likely to exhibit delusional beliefs and to show a more rapid decline of cognitive function. Psychotic symptoms are associated with problem behaviours such as agitation and wandering. These contribute most to carer distress and increase the likelihood of admission to hospital or placement into residential or nursing home care.

SLEEP AND APPETITE DISTURBANCE

3.24 What patterns of sleep disturbance occur in dementia?

An important feature of dementia is the disturbance of the sleep/wake cycle. Patients often rise in the early hours, believing it to be morning. They might dress and attempt to leave the house as if departing for work. Conversely, they might sleep for long periods during the day, becoming disorientated on awaking. Many patients with dementia go through phases of wakefulness during both day and night. This is typically associated with wandering or pacing. Disturbance of sleep pattern is a prominent feature of dementia with Lewy bodies.

When dementia is associated with depression or anxiety, other disturbances of the sleep pattern might be seen, such as initial insomnia where the patient tosses and turns for hours before settling to sleep. Alternatively, early morning waking is seen in depression.

3.25 Do appetite changes occur in patients with dementia?

Many patients experience a diminished appetite as they get older. Patients with dementia might lose their appetite and weight loss in the later stages is almost inevitable. Others refuse food, perhaps in response to the abnormal belief that is being poisoned.

Patients who have lost the ability to feed themselves, or have difficulty swallowing, should not be assumed to have lost their appetite. Also, patients who pace the floor might not be able to sit still for long enough to eat conventionally, and will lose weight. Imaginative and flexible methods of providing nutrition become necessary.

Many patients, and particularly those with front lobe dementia, develop a 'sweet tooth' (*see Q 12.8*). The Kluver Bucy syndrome – whereby a patient overeats, binges or ingests inedible objects – occurs not just in dementias but also in tumours or strokes affecting parts of the temporal lobes or limbic system.

BEHAVIOURAL DISTURBANCE AND PERSONALITY CHANGE

3.26 What changes to motor activity are seen in dementia?

Wandering, pacing and restlessness are common in dementia. Various studies have identified prevalences of between 20 and 60%. There are many causes of wandering and attempts should be made to identify them. Such behaviour might be associated with repetitive semipurposeful activity, such as attempts at housework. Other causes include pain or discomfort, boredom or depression. Repeated attempts to leave the house are often due to profound disorientation; patients often state that they must be 'getting to work' or need to 'go home'.

Another important cause of restlessness and agitation is medication. Neuroleptics, such as haloperidol, which might be prescribed with the intention of calming agitation, sometimes cause motor and psychological restlessness (akathisia). They can also worsen agitation by causing extrapyramidal symptoms, including tremor.

Not all patients wander; some become lethargic, apathetic and lacking in motivation and drive. In these circumstances it is necessary to exclude depression, and a trial of antidepressants should be considered.

3.27 What is 'agitation'?

Agitation is a poorly defined term. It is usually taken to mean inappropriate motor, verbal or vocal activity. Examples of motor behaviour include repetitive, purposeless movements including pacing, hand wringing, foot tapping, fiddling with hair, clothes or other objects. Vocal agitation includes repetitive utterances, groaning and shouting.

3.28 Apart from dementia, what other factors are associated with agitation?

Agitation can be predicted in patients with dementia who are also depressed, anxious or who are in physical discomfort or pain (*Box 3.1*). Environmental factors associated with physical discomfort include isolation

> **Box 3.1 Some causes of restlessness or agitation in dementia**
> ■ Boredom
> ■ Frustration
> ■ Isolation
> ■ Overstimulation
> ■ Depression
> ■ Physical discomfort or pain
> ■ Side-effects of medication
> ■ Delirium

or overstimulation (a noisy and overcrowded day room for instance). Frustration over communication difficulties often results in agitation. Delirium should be considered when a known patient with dementia suddenly becomes agitated.

Verbal agitation is more common in women than in men and has been shown to be particularly related to higher levels of pain, physical illness and a poor quality of relationship with staff.

3.29 What is 'sundowning'?

Sundowning is the commonly observed phenomenon of an increase in agitation and worsening disorientation in patients with dementia as the evening draws in. One explanation is that the clarity of visual cues worsens as it becomes darker. However, it also occurs in well-lit environments, suggesting an abnormality in the patient's circadian rhythm or sleep cycle. Tiredness at the end of the day might also be a factor.

3.30 What is 'disinhibition'?

Disinhibition in this context means the loss of emotional or behavioural control. A patient might become more short tempered and less considerate of others. Verbal abuse, swearing or aggression can result.

3.31 What changes to sexual behaviour occur in dementia?

In general, sexual behaviour within an established relationship is diminished where one of the couple has dementia. This might be due to loss of libido or erectile dysfunction, which appears to be relatively common in men with Alzheimer's disease. However, an increased demand for intercourse might occur due to loss of memory or loss of social control. Conversely, the strain of caring might lead to a reduction in libido on the part of a spouse. Clearly all these scenarios can place an even greater strain on a relationship.

Abnormally increased sexual behaviour typically occurs in dementia associated with frontal lobe damage. Sexual disinhibition takes various forms, from socially inappropriate use of sexual language, propositioning or innuendo through to exposing of genitals or masturbation in public, and touching others in a sexual manner. Such behaviour is a particular problem in residential care settings where patients live in close proximity to relative strangers (of both genders) and where young and inexperienced female care workers provide intimate personal care. Unfortunately, this also frequently results in a lack of tolerance of normal expressions of sexuality (see *www.dementiacare.org.uk* for information on understanding and managing sexual activity amongst patients with dementia).

3.32 When does personality change occur?

Personality change occurs to some extent in most cases of dementia. In some forms, notably the frontotemporal dementias, changes in personality or social behaviour can be the presenting feature before cognitive decline becomes apparent. By contrast, in Alzheimer's disease and vascular dementia, personality can remain relatively well preserved until later on in the course of the illness. Such change might be the emergence of new personality traits or the exaggeration of those that existed before the onset of dementia. These traits include apathy, irritability, indifference, disinhibition, belligerence and euphoria.

3.33 What is the impact of behavioural or personality change on carers?

It is frequently behavioural disturbance, rather than cognitive impairment, that carers find stressful. Night-time disruption leading to loss of sleep is an important factor, as are verbal or physical aggression, sexual disinhibition and incontinence. Loss of privacy resulting from not being able to separate, even briefly, from a dependent spouse is also extremely stressful, irrespective of the quality of the marital relationship.

PATIENT QUESTIONS

3.34 I am always having to remind my husband to eat and drink. Does it matter?

Changes in appetite are very common in patients with dementia and loss of weight is common. Maintaining good physical health is as important for people with dementia as for anyone else and a balanced diet with plenty of fruit and vegetables is recommended. This might well help prevent constipation that can aggravate agitation or confusion in patients with dementia. A diet lacking in calcium and other minerals can make the bones more brittle and increase the risk of fractures. Lack of vitamins and protein will lower the ability to fight infection and affect wound healing. Patients need to drink plenty of fluid because dehydration causes constipation and will also worsen the confusion.

3.35 My mother has started accusing me of stealing her belongings. This is upsetting me, why is she doing this?

Poor memory will result in your mother mislaying her belongings, and problems in recognising objects means that things will often get put away in the wrong places. She might not realize that she has problems, so rather than accepting she has misplaced something your mother jumps to the conclusion that it has been stolen. She might then try to hide valuables (so that they aren't stolen) and then later be unable to find them. This, in her mind, confirms her belief. If you are the person who visits most often then you might well be the one she accuses.

Reversible causes of dementia

4

4.1 Are there treatable causes of dementia?

One of the major tasks of the physician seeing a new patient with dementia is to exclude the treatable causes. This is usually a straightforward task – the combination of a typical clinical profile of Alzheimer's disease or vascular dementia plus a normal CT or MRI scan is usually sufficient. Physicians and psychiatrists do see a steady trickle of patients with a treatable underlying condition presenting with cognitive problems. By far the most common treatable cause of cognitive problems is depression, which is dealt with in Chapter 3.

4.2 What are the treatable dementias?

A large number of dementias are potentially treatable. They can be divided into those that need surgical treatment and those that need medical treatment (*Box 4.1*).

Box 4.1 More common treatable dementias

Surgically treated dementias:
- Normal pressure hydrocephalus
- Brain tumours
- Meningiomas
- Subdural haematomas
- Hydrocephalus

Medically treated dementias:
- Hypothyroidism
- HIV infection
- Alcohol abuse
- Vitamin B_{12} deficiency
- Chronic hypoxia, e.g. from obstructive sleep apnoea or neuromuscular disease
- Cerebral vasculitis
- Virtually any metabolic or endocrine disturbance
- Neurosyphilis
- Other CNS infections
- Hashimoto's encephalopathy
- Wilson's disease
- Chronic meningoencephalitis
- Coeliac disease
- Whipple's disease

4.3 How common are treatable dementias?

Approximately 1 in 10 patients with dementia have a treatable cause (*Box 4.2*). The proportion of patients with a treatable dementia seen by a particular doctor varies according to the referral pattern. Patients with treatable causes for their cognitive problems often have rapid progression of their problems, with focal neurological signs and abnormal brain scans. They will therefore tend to present acutely to neurologists, accident and emergency departments and physicians rather than to memory clinics.

Only a tiny proportion of patients with a long history of dementia and a pattern of problems typical of Alzheimer's disease will have a treatable cause of dementia. It is quite possible for physicians or psychiatrists to spend their working lives seeing patients with a clinical diagnosis of typical Alzheimer's disease, not arrange imaging and not miss a treatable dementia as a result. Patients presenting with a frontotemporal dementia have a much higher chance of having a treatable cause for their dementia and most should have a CT or MRI scan.

Box 4.2 The common potentially treatable 'dementias' (listed in order of frequency)
- Depression
- Hydrocephalus
- Alcohol abuse
- Tumours
- Seizures
- Thyroid disease
- Vitamin B_{12} deficiency

NORMAL PRESSURE HYDROCEPHALUS (NPH)

4.4 What is hydrocephalus?

There is normally a free flow of cerebrospinal fluid (CSF) within the ventricles in the centre of the brain and between the ventricles and the surface of the brain and spinal cord. Blockage of the flow of CSF in the ventricular system usually occurs in the third or fourth ventricles (including its outflow) and gives rise to obstructive hydrocephalus. This usually presents acutely with headaches, vomiting and mental dulling. The causes of obstructive hydrocephalus include tumours and bleeds in the posterior fossa.

Some causes of obstructive hydrocephalus are less dramatic and patients born with a narrowing of the third ventricle (called congenital aqueduct stenosis) might present in middle life with mental dulling and gait disturbance.

There are less dramatic forms of hydrocephalus; poor absorption of the cerebrospinal fluid or partial blockage can lead to a communicating hydrocephalus in which the pressure of the fluid is raised although the ventricular output is still patent. Communicating hydrocephalus leads to gradual dilatation of the ventricles and a subacute syndrome of gait and memory problems.

At one end of the spectrum of communicating hydrocephalus lies normal pressure hydrocephalus (NPH). In NPH, the pressure within the ventricles is raised intermittently, with pulses of high pressure every few hours. A single pressure measurement is therefore usually normal. The name 'normal pressure' hydrocephalus is confusing and wrong. If the pressure is monitored over a day or more then waves of increased pressure are seen from time to time. The clinical features of NPH evolve over months. The intermittent increased pressure leads to slow dilatation of the ventricles and increasing disability.

Headaches and papilloedema are not features of NPH.

4.5   What are the features of NPH?

NPH is a rare disease of middle life and old age. Many patients will have had a previous neurological problem, such as a subarachnoid haemorrhage or bacterial meningitis, which led to the problems with CSF flow and absorption resulting in the NPH. A triad of features characterizes NPH:

- ■ slowing of cognition
- ■ incontinence and frequency of micturition
- ■ a slow, stiff, unsteady gait.

Patients with a presumptive but incorrect diagnosis of NPH are often referred to neurologists and memory clinics. The usual scenario is that a CT brain scan has been performed in a patient suspected of having a degenerative or vascular dementia and the patient has been referred because the radiologist's report suggests NPH. It is important to assess whether this diagnosis is correct as some patients with NPH (*see Q 4.8*) respond well to treatment that involves shunting the enlarged ventricles. However, shunting the ventricles is not a benign procedure and has a number of complications, particularly in the elderly. If patients without NPH (e.g. those with Alzheimer's disease and vascular dementia, who share some features with NPH) are shunted then harm will be done through the development of surgical complications such as subdural haematomas and shunt infections.

4.6 How are cognition, urinary problems and gait problems assessed in NPH?

COGNITION

It is important to assess whether the patient has any of the specific problems with cognition that suggest cortical damage, or if there is a general slowing and dysexecutive syndrome suggesting a subcortical dementia. The typical patient with NPH is apathetic and slow, and finds it difficult to plan complex tasks.

The difference between subcortical and cortical dementias is discussed in *Question 14.9*. Specific cortical deficits, such as nominal aphasia and alexia, suggest that the patient has cortical disease, and hence a degenerative dementia and not NPH.

URINARY FREQUENCY AND INCONTINENCE

There are many more common causes of urinary frequency and incontinence than NPH and it is important to screen for these first. Dementia and urinary problems are both common in the elderly and will therefore often present together by chance. However, degenerative dementias are also a cause of urinary problems – incontinence is a feature of frontal lobe dementias.

The typical incontinence of NPH occurs without warning, the patient might be unconcerned about the problem.

GAIT

Gait is the aspect most likely to improve following shunting for NPH. Evaluation of the gait is therefore an important part of the assessment of possible NPH. Gait problems, like urinary and cognitive problems, are common in the elderly. The typical gait of NPH is slow and apraxic. Patients have difficulty starting to walk and are very unsteady and slow to walk. They take short steps. Rising from a chair and starting to walk is particularly slow. By contrast, on the bed the legs seem to work well and there are no obvious signs of Parkinson's disease or pyramidal weakness. When asked to mime walking or cycling on the bed, patients can generally move the legs surprisingly well. Gait problems are easily overlooked if the patient is not seen walking or can be dismissed as non-organic because of the normality of the examination on the bed.

The most common cause of an apraxic gait is small vessel disease.

4.7 Which investigations should be done in suspected NPH?

The initial investigation is usually a CT scan, which is an important investigation because the clinical picture of NPH can be mimicked by a frontal tumour or obstructive hydrocephalus. A typical patient with NPH has enlargement of the lateral ventricles without significant superficial cortical atrophy. There is no evidence of strokes and little periventricular white matter changes. A MRI scan usually provides additional information, such as white matter changes and radiological 'strokes', which are not visible on the CT scan. The presence of white matter changes around the ventricle raises the possibility of small vessels disease. If there are subcortical white matter changes these are likely to be vascular and predict a poor response to surgery.

If there is a high suspicion of NPH, the patient should be referred to a neurologist or neurosurgeon. Removal of 15–20 mL CSF via a lumbar puncture sometimes leads to a dramatic improvement in a timed walk and strengthens the case for shunting. As the CSF reforms within hours, the timed walk must be done immediately. However, no response to the removal of CSF does not exclude NPH. It is often necessary to do more invasive tests with intracranial or lumbar pressure monitoring.

4.8 Which patients with possible NPH should be referred for shunting?

In the past, many patients were shunted for normal pressure hydrocephalus. However, the complications that ensued and the low success rate led to a reappraisal and now comparatively few operations are done. The following are criteria to assess the likelihood of success with surgery:

- a clear cause for the NPH, such as a history of meningitis or subarachnoid haemorrhage, which has led to partial blockage of CSF flow or reduced reabsorption
- if the major problem is the apraxic gait and the patient is cognitively well preserved
- if removal of 20–30 mL CSF leads to a measurable improvement (such as in a timed walk) in the gait
- the absence of vascular risk factors and no evidence of vascular disease on CT or MRI scanning
- a short progressive history; if the patient's walking distance is rapidly reducing week by week then this is a strong indicator for surgery.

If a patient's problems are static or improving then surgery is usually not indicated. Sometimes it is useful to monitor patients medically for a period. If there is a clear deterioration then the argument for surgery is strengthened.

4.9 What are the results of shunting for NPH?

Controlled trials are not available. Anecdotally, many patients do very well with shunting provided they are selected carefully. Unfortunately, shunting cognitively impaired elderly patients can result in such problems as subdural haematoma, shunt blockages and infections, all of which can make the patient's condition far worse than it was before the shunt. The hazards of shunting and the frequency with which patients are seen with memory problems together with mild gait and urinary problems reinforces the need for careful selection of patients for shunting. The clinical features, and in particular the history of the deterioration and the nature and severity of the gait problems, are the crucial factors in deciding who to refer; the appearance of the CT scan is less important.

4.10 Do other forms of hydrocephalus cause dementia?

Yes. Any form of hydrocephalus can cause cognitive problems. Hydrocephalus often presents acutely, with the patient developing a severe headache and progressive deterioration in level of consciousness over a few hours or days. Milder forms of hydrocephalus can present more gradually with slowing of intellect and gait problems. If the hydrocephalus is obstructive then patients will usually be referred to a neurosurgeon for consideration of shunting.

Patients with communicating hydrocephalus need more careful assessment. The underlying cause – most commonly congenital aqueduct stenosis – is often not progressive. The clinical history and the radiological appearances are the crucial factors in determining the correct treatment. A static history and a scan showing chronic hydrocephalus usually result in conservative treatment.

VITAMIN B₁₂ DEFICIENCY DEMENTIA

4.11 What are the features of vitamin B$_{12}$ deficiency dementia?

Vitamin B$_{12}$ deficiency causes an encephalopathy with a progressive amnesia and drowsiness coupled with apathy and limb problems. The limb problems are due to associated subacute combined degeneration of the spinal cord. The initial problem is unpleasant pins and needles often starting in the hands and later spreading to the legs. Patients sometimes note that flexion of the neck causes shocks down the spine. This is called Lhermitte's phenomenon (it is more often a feature of multiple sclerosis). If not treated, the symptoms develop and patients develop irreversible dementia plus myelopathy and peripheral neuropathy. On examination, patients are apathetic and slow. They have loss of joint-position sense in the hands and feet, pyramidal signs in the legs with increased tone and pyramidal weakness coupled with sensory changes, absent ankle jerks and extensor plantars.

Full-blown neurological vitamin B$_{12}$ deficiency is very rare now. A far more common problem is the patient with a typical degenerative dementia who has a mildly low B$_{12}$ level. In such patients, the low B$_{12}$

is probably irrelevant – especially if there is no other evidence of B_{12} deficiency (such as red cell macrocytosis). However, B_{12} replacement is straightforward and very unlikely to do any harm, and it is therefore sensible to investigate and treat such patients for vitamin B_{12} deficiency.

4.12 Can a patient with a normal haemoglobin and red cell size still develop neurological problems because of vitamin B_{12} deficiency?

The short answer is yes. Most cases of neurological vitamin B_{12} deficiency have a macrocytosis and an anaemia but there are cases where the haematological indices are normal. The serum B_{12} is also very low in most patients who have neurological disease secondary to B_{12} deficiency.

Occasionally, subacute combined degeneration of the cord is precipitated iatrogenically when a patient with vitamin B_{12} deficiency is treated with folate.

4.13 How do you manage vitamin B_{12} deficiency dementia?

Vitamin B_{12} deficiency needs to be investigated. The cause is nearly always poor absorption of the vitamin, for example as a result of pernicious anaemia. Vitamin B_{12} needs to be replaced parenterally. It is usual to replenish diminished stores of vitamin B_{12} by giving 1 mg every 1–3 days intramuscularly until 7–12 doses have been given. The maintenance therapy is 1 mg hydroxycobalamin intramuscularly once every 3 months. The patient should be referred to a haematologist to find and treat the cause of the deficiency.

TUMOURS AND DEMENTIA

4.14 What tumours cause dementia?

Virtually any brain tumour can cause dementia. Tumours usually present subacutely. They can present in patients with a degenerative dementia and the appearance of unusual features, such as a rapid onset of mutism, is a reason to image. *Figure 4.1* shows a left frontal metastasis and mild hydrocephalus in a patient with mild long-standing amnesia who then became a mute.

Tumours cause dementia through direct effects on the brain, through swelling of brain tissue or if the tumour is below the tentorium through hydrocephalus. The tumours that classically mimic a degenerative dementia are frontal meningiomas. Non-dominant frontal meningiomas can grow to a large size and cause minimal effects apart from a mild frontal dementia. The presentation of such tumours is with personality change, apathy and a dysexecutive syndrome. Focal neurological signs are unusual, although there might be a unilateral grasp reflex or extensor plantar response. A classic physical sign associated with frontal meningiomas is loss of smell, but there are many more common causes of this. If the frontal tumour is undetected it will eventually cause an expressive aphasia (on the dominant side) or a contralateral hemiparesis affecting the leg more than the arm. Occasionally, meningiomas are found during investigation of late-onset epilepsy.

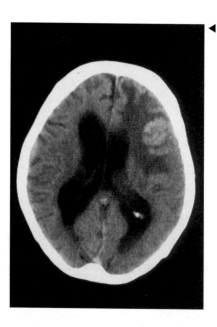

Fig. 4.1 Left frontal lobe tumour (metastasis) and mild hydrocephalus shown on a CT scan in an 84-year-old patient with long-standing mild memory problems and recent loss of speech.

4.15 What features suggest that a patient with dementia has a cerebral tumour?

The usual features that suggest a tumour are:

- onset over a few days or weeks
- seizures (can occur in Alzheimer's disease and vascular dementia)

- focal signs such as a hemianopia or hemiplegia (very often on the dominant side)
- features of raised intracranial pressure – postural headache, vomiting, papilloedema.

4.16 Are tumours that cause dementia operable?

This depends largely on whether they are tumours of the brain substance itself – usually gliomas, which cannot be cured by surgery – or tumours of the coverings of the brain – meningiomas, which can often be removed. Tumours that cause dementia are usually large, which makes surgery more complex. Other treatments such as radiotherapy might be appropriate.

OTHER CAUSES OF DEMENTIA

4.17 Does coeliac disease cause dementia?

It is very rare for coeliac disease to cause a dementia but it does occasionally cause brain disease, which can occur in patients with known coeliac disease or be a presenting feature. The typical picture is a combination of a mild encephalopathy with myoclonus and seizures. Brain disease can occur with other features of coeliac disease, such as diarrhoea and weight loss, or without them. It can be screened for serologically by testing for antigliadin antibodies, followed by a jejunal biopsy if positive. A red cell macrocytosis is a clue. MRI scan might be normal or show non-specific white-matter changes; CSF might show a mild increase in white cells. Coeliac disease is treated with a gluten-free diet; there are reports of improvement with steroids.

4.18 What is Whipple's disease?

Whipple's disease is a bowel disease caused by a mycobacterium-like organism and often presents with diarrhoea and weight loss. It can cause a large number of neurological problems, although each is very rare. It can cause a dementia/encephalopathy, often with a movement disorder of the eyes and jaw. The MRI usually shows disease of the white and grey matter. Diagnosis is usually made by duodenal or other biopsy, although new genetic techniques can help, for example using the polymerase chain reaction to amplify the organism's DNA from the spinal fluid. It is treated with prolonged courses of antibiotics.

4.19 What are the features of neurosyphilis?

Neurosyphilis in patients with a normal immune system has now become extremely rare. Early syphilis infections – so-called primary syphilis – still occur and the rarity of the later neurosyphilis is probably a result of the number of courses of antibiotics patients now receive for other reasons, which incidentally kill the trepenomes that cause syphilis. The time between primary syphilis and neurosyphilis used to be 10 or more years – allowing plenty of time for incidental antibiotics to be effective.

Neurosyphilis is famous for the many ways in which it can present. The two main types of neurosyphilis that affect the brain are:

- Neurovascular syphilis, which presents with strokes. These are often multiple and tend to affect the posterior circulation of the brain, producing diplopia, vertigo, dysarthria and clumsiness.
- General paralysis of the insane (GPI), which presents with a combination of a frontal lobe dementia with personality change and spinal cord disease causing weakness of the legs and loss of joint position sense in the legs that results in a stamping gait when the patient tries to walk. Patients with GPI often confabulate and have features of other forms of neurosyphilis, such as small, irregular pupils that react to accommodation but not to light (Argyll Robertson pupils).

4.20 What investigations help the diagnosis of neurosyphilis?

The initial screening test for neurosyphilis is a VDRL/TPHA. The VDRL (Venereal Disease Reference Laboratory test) is sensitive to trepenome infection but not specific. The TPHA (*Trepenoma pallidum* haemagglutination test) is relatively specific but less sensitive. If both these are positive then the patient is very likely to have had a trepenomal infection. However, as other trepenomal infections, such as Yaws (which affects people of Caribbean origin) are not uncommon, more specific tests need to be performed. Tests such as the FTA (fixed trepenome haemagglutination test) are suggestive of active infection. The most important test is to perform a lumbar puncture and see if there is evidence of trepenomal infection of the CNS. The features of CNS infection in the CSF are:

- a positive VDRL
- increased protein and white cells
- oligoclonal bands.

4.21 What is the treatment of neurosyphilis?

Once proven, neurosyphilis should be treated with a 4-week course of antibiotics. Intravenous benzyl penicillin is the best treatment. Alternatives include intramuscular penicillin plus probenecid and doxycyline.

4.22 Can other infections cause dementia?

The most common infection that causes a dementia is human immunodeficiency virus (HIV; *see Q 4.23*).

Patients with a subacute dementia and an active CSF, or other sign of infection, need to be screened for infections; syphilis, acquired immunodeficiency syndrome (Aids), tuberculosis, Lyme disease, cryptococcus and Whipple's disease can present in this way.

4.23 What are the features of HIV-associated dementia?

HIV infection can cause a dementia through direct infection of the CNS by the HIV virus. It can also produce dementia through:

■ other CNS infections
■ cerebral tumours
■ progressive multifocal leukoencephalopathy (discussed in Chapter 14).

HIV infection is a very rare presentation to memory clinics but it can be the first manifestation of Aids.

The typical presentation is with a combination of apathy and amnesia. The diagnosis is usually straightforward if the patient is known to have Aids. The development of other manifestations of Aids – both neurological and non-neurological – provides further clues. Structural imaging reveals cerebral atrophy with or without white matter changes and the CSF findings are typical of those seen in chronic infections, with a mild increase in white cells and protein and oligoclonal bands. Aids is treated by HAART (highly active anti-retroviral therapy).

4.24 What are the features of hypothyroid dementia?

These days, with the wide availability of thyroid testing, a frank dementia due to hypothyroidism is very rare. Patients generally have other features of hypothyroidism, such as weight gain, slowing and skin changes. If untreated, patients can become comatose. Other presentations include slowing of mentation with apathy. Some present with forgetfulness.

Because thyroid disease is treatable, hypothyroidism should be considered in every patient presenting with dementia. Hypothyroid disease is treated by cautious replacement of the missing hormone, thyroxine. Established cases of hypothyroid dementia might be only partially responsive to treatment, so early diagnosis is important.

4.25 What other metabolic causes of dementia need to be considered?

Most endocrine and metabolic diseases can cause cognitive problems. If the metabolic disorder occurs subacutely the patient often presents with an encephalopathy – with a reduced level of consciousness and myoclonus (including the so-called liver flap). The most common causes of metabolic encephalopathy are renal failure, liver failure and respiratory failure. These can be screened for with blood tests including urea, electrolytes, liver function and arterial blood gases.

In more chronic conditions, the presentation can be more subtle, with a less specific deterioration in motivation and cognition. Other possible causes of metabolic encephalopathies include alterations in the blood calcium and sodium. The treatment is usually to treat the underlying condition; in hepatic encephalopathy there are specific measures to try to reduce the encephalopathy.

4.26 Which drugs cause dementia?

 A large number of drugs cause cognitive side-effects, a few can produce a dementia. Some produce a dementia as a rare metabolic side-effect in susceptible individuals. Valproate occasionally produces dementia associated with elevated plasma ammonia levels. This seems to be more common in patients with underlying neurological disease, such as cerebral palsy, and a plasma ammonia level should be considered in such patients who are deteriorating cognitively.

Other drugs can cause a chronic dementia that usually improves with withdrawal of the drug. It has been described with the following drugs:

- phenobarbitone and other barbiturates
- lithium
- phenytoin
- opiates.

4.27 What is Hashimoto's encephalopathy?

Hashimoto's encephalopathy is a newly described and unusual disease. It occurs in individuals of all ages. There is often a history of autoimmune thyroid disease. The presentation is with a subacute encephalopathy with a fluctuating level of consciousness. It can be associated with hypo- or hyperthyroidism but most cases are euthyroid. There is often myoclonus or seizures. Imaging with CT scan or MRI might be normal or can show white matter changes and the EEG suggests an encephalopathy. The CSF often contains a small excess of lymphocytes and there might be oligoclonal bands in CSF and/or serum. The diagnosis is made by the combination of the clinical features and high titres of thyroid microsomal antibodies in the serum.

The condition responds well to corticosteroids. These are usually given as high-dose IV methyl prednisolone followed by a reducing oral dose.

4.28 What features suggest a cerebral vasculitis?

Cerebral vasculitis is a rare condition that can be hard to diagnose and hard to treat. There are two forms:

■ a cerebral vasculitis that occurs as part of a systemic vasculitis when the patient has evidence of systemic disease affecting the skin, kidney, joints, heart, etc.
■ an isolated cerebral vasculitis.

The usual presentation of cerebral problems is with multiple strokes occurring over a few days or weeks. There is often fever and headache and, if there is a systemic vasculitis, features such as Raynaud's phenomenon, nail-fold infarcts, dusky fingers arthralgias/arthritis, renal failure, mononeuritis multiplex and rashes. Some patients have a more gradual presentation of their problems over a few months. Typically, the disease runs a very aggressive course.

4.29 What investigations should be considered in cerebral vasculitis?

Extensive investigations are often needed:

■ Serological tests should include: autoantibody screen, antiphospholipid antibodies, anti-ds DNA antibodies, antineutrophil cytoplasmic antibodies (ANCA), erythrocyte sedimentation rate (ESR) and C-reactive protein (CRP).
■ CT/MRI scanning can show distinct infarcts or more confluent grey- and white-matter lesions.
■ CSF usually shows a polymorphic leukocytosis with increased protein and oligoclonal bands.
■ Cerebral angiography is usually normal but can show a distinctive beading appearance of small arteries, which is diagnostic.
■ Cerebral biopsy is often needed but might not be diagnostic.

The common systemic disorders associated with a cerebral vasculitis include systemic lupus erythematosus (SLE), polyarteritis nodosa, Wegener's granulomatosis. Vasculitis can also occur with a variety of other diseases and can be associated with infections and tumours.

4.30 How is cerebral vasculitis treated?

The usual treatment for cerebral vasculitis is a combination of corticosteroids and immunosuppresive therapy with cyclophosphamide or a similar agent. The initial treatment is usually high-dose IV corticosteroids;

less toxic immunosuppressants seem to be less effective. The deterioration in cerebral vasculitis is often sudden and might not reverse with treatment. This, combined with the lack of a peripheral marker to monitor the progress of the disease, makes titrating treatment very difficult. Relapses are usually treated with IV steroids or IV immunoglobulin.

4.31 What are the features of chronic subdural haematoma?

A unilateral subdural haematoma usually produces a combination of headache, mental slowing and a gradually progressive hemiplegia; bilateral subdurals can present in less obvious ways. Bilateral subdurals also tend to occur in the very elderly or in alcoholics – both groups that can be assumed to have other, more common, causes for their problems. There might be a history of head trauma but often there is not (either it was trivial or has been forgotten). The usual presentation is with a progressive slowing of thought and mild obtundation accompanied by 'going off their legs'. On examination, some patients have papilloedema, which should prompt an urgent CT scan. Other patients have some evidence of pyramidal tract disease, such as bilateral extensor plantar responses, but have an apraxic gait (*see Q 2.8*); diagnosis is by CT or MRI scanning.

Occasionally, bilateral subdural haematomas are seen in patients with general slowing and no hard physical signs.

The treatment is surgical drainage but conservative treatment is sometimes preferred. If the patient is asymptomatic or improving then there is usually no need for surgery. The major problem of surgical drainage is the recurrence of the subdurals – sometimes causing more problems than the original ones.

Non-pharmacological management of dementia

5

PQ PATIENT QUESTIONS

5.1   What are the main principles of dementia care?

One of the important developments in dementia care over the last decade has been that of person-centred care. This is the philosophy of care that emphasizes the fact that the patient with dementia remains an adult human being with rights, wishes, hopes and fears. It is the duty of all who work with patients with dementia always to respect these.

Appropriate management of dementia starts with diagnosis. Ensuring that necessary information and advice is provided is a vital part of the early encounters with patient and carers. Subsequent involvement depends on circumstances and clinical need. Medication, psychological therapies, behaviour management techniques and continuing emotional and practical support all carry potential benefit. There might be specific drug treatment that can be offered. Even if there is, other forms of intervention or treatment are likely to be equally relevant, less likely to cause harm and should not be neglected. Where no drug treatment is indicated it is important not to assume that 'nothing can be done' and retreat into therapeutic nihilism.

Assistance with personal care and protection from harm are important aspects of care. But this becomes dehumanized and mechanical when viewed in isolation, away from a consideration of the person behind the condition. In recent years there has been a positive move towards encouraging independence, optimizing functioning and accepting that patients with dementia are individuals in their own right. For all who are involved in the care of people with dementia, this entails ensuring their dignity, considering their needs, likes and dislikes and respecting them as adults.

5.2   What are the main aims in managing dementia?

The main aims of dementia management can be summarized as follows:

- ■ identify and treat, if possible, the cause of the dementia
- ■ manage or treat coexisting illness
- ■ identify, try to understand and tackle each major problem of behaviour
- ■ identify and minimize risk
- ■ involve and support the carer(s) throughout.

DISCLOSURE OF DIAGNOSIS

5.3   How much should I tell the patient about the diagnosis?

Before any specific management can be contemplated, the patient and carers need information about the condition. Doctors are sometimes reluctant to disclose the diagnosis of dementia because they believe that 'nothing can be done', or are perhaps asked by relatives to withhold the diagnosis so as not to distress the patient unnecessarily. In many ways this was the situation with cancer 20 years ago. Now, most people would accept that patients with cancer should be informed of the diagnosis, even if no active treatment is possible.

With dementia, however, there are three additional difficulties. One is the stigma associated with the condition. The second is that bad news, having been broken, can soon be forgotten. Finally, diagnosis in the early stages might not be clear. For whatever reason, the majority of GPs are unlikely to fully disclose a diagnosis of dementia to a patient; old-age psychiatrists are not always much better.

Recent research indicates that although relatives might prefer their affected loved ones not to know, the majority of these same relatives would themselves wish to be informed if they were in a similar predicament. The general principle, therefore, should be that most patients should be made aware – with appropriate tact and sensitivity – of their diagnosis. But with diagnosis must come information, not only about the illness but also about local services available to help the sufferer and carer.

As with discussions about other serious illnesses, it is necessary to judge how much detail should be disclosed and at what speed; the process of disclosure might need to be taken gradually. In many cases the patient will take the lead by asking for information, having already guessed the diagnosis. On the other hand, if the disease is severe there might be little to be gained from a formal discussion of the diagnosis.

5.4 Families are often worried about the distress caused, so what are the benefits of telling patients their diagnosis?

Most would agree that patients have the right to receive information about their condition, even if this causes them distress. The need for accurate and prompt diagnosis and disclosure of diagnosis has become greater since the introduction of specific drugs for Alzheimer's disease. Prescription and the necessary monitoring cannot be done without first having discussed the diagnosis with both patient and carer.

Knowing the diagnosis and the likely progression of the disease can also encourage patients to get their financial affairs in order, make a will, and so on, to ensure that relatives are properly provided for in the future. For example, an enduring power of attorney must be organized before the patient loses the capacity to do this. Early disclosure of diagnosis will allow both patient and carer to receive advice and support before a crisis occurs. It also enables the issue of driving safety to be addressed properly.

PSYCHOLOGICAL TREATMENTS IN DEMENTIA

5.5   What psychological interventions can be used in dementia?

A range of psychological approaches can be used in patients with dementia. These include simple reassurance and emotional support, which will be particularly beneficial when combined with the provision of practical support and information. Anxiety management techniques or relaxation training can help distressed patients with early dementia. Anxious carers would also benefit.

Various psychological methods can be used to reduce the frequency or severity of challenging behaviours. One example is the use of operant conditioning (rewards and reinforcements) to reduce aggressive or 'attention-seeking' behaviour in a residential care setting (*see Q 5.15*).

Other techniques are used to reduce patients' distress by aiming to improve their awareness of their environment, facilitating communication and encouraging recall and discussion of remembered significant events.

5.6   What is reality orientation?

This aims to improve patients' orientation and awareness of their environment through a variety of prompts and activities. At a very basic level this could mean a carer providing reminders of the date, location, and so on during everyday conversation. Calendars and clocks in prominent positions and signs on doors will also help orientation. In a more structured setting, such as in a home or hospital ward, in addition to verbal prompts and noticeboards with details of the date and weather, there could be regular discussion groups designed to enhance awareness of what is happening around them. There is some evidence that this technique improves orientation, communication and behaviour. However, it can cause distress if used insensitively; unpleasant reality should not be 'forced' on a patient.

5.7   What is validation therapy?

Reality orientation emphasizes the 'here and now' and can be rather mechanical. By contrast, validation therapy recognizes the importance of the patients' feelings and their attempts to express them. Rather than correcting factual errors in a conversation, the aim is to seek the meanings behind verbal and non-verbal communication and to gain an empathetic understanding of the individual. For example, instead of correcting a patient who anxiously expresses a hope that a (long dead) parent will be visiting soon, a nurse might use the patient's anxiety to address issues of loneliness, insecurity and family relationships. Although there is little objective evidence that this approach improves 'outcome', it is likely to be beneficial from a humanitarian point of view because it encourages staff to consider the emotional as well as the practical consequences of dementia. Carers and family members can also be encouraged to use this approach.

5.8 What is reminiscence therapy?

Reminiscence therapy encourages recollections of details or events in an individual's life. It can be done individually or in a group setting. Prompts such as appropriate music or photographs are used to trigger discussion. Reminiscence, in turn, can facilitate a more in-depth review of a patient's life. This technique allows carers to gain a much greater insight into their patients' backgrounds and to see beyond the dementia. The quality of the carers' contact with the patient will be enhanced as a result.

BEHAVIOURAL PROBLEMS IN DEMENTIA

5.9 How do I identify problem behaviours?

There are three main groups of problem behaviour:

- lack of behaviour: patients do not seem to function as well as they are capable of doing, e.g. they decline to get out of bed, refuse to socialize with others, will not feed without assistance
- behaviour might be an exaggerated form of normal functioning, such as wandering
- abnormal and undesirable behaviour, such as extreme sexual disinhibition.

5.10 What are the main examples of problem behaviours?

- Restlessness and agitation, including pacing, wandering.
- Irritability, including verbal or physical aggression.
- Lack of cooperation with care.
- Urinary incontinence, including micturating in inappropriate locations.
- Sleep disturbance, including change to the sleep/wake cycle.
- Dietary change, including loss of appetite and bingeing.
- Sexual disinhibition, ranging from flirting to masturbating in public.

5.11 How do I understand problem behaviours?

Problem behaviours often have many possible causes, not all of which are to do with the patients themselves.

'Urinary incontinence' can be due to loss of bladder control or infection. Alternatively, poor mobility might mean that the patient cannot reach the toilet in time. Or the dementia might be such that the patient cannot find the toilet or does not recognize it for what it is. Patients might feel a sense of shame that young female carers must assist with toileting. Or the 'incontinence' might simply be due to inadequate signs on the toilet doors.

'Loss of appetite' might be due to depression or physical ill health, or because the patient is unable to reach the tray of food placed at the end of the bed. Patients might also be offered food that they dislike and therefore leave.

'Wandering' can be the result of anxiety, the search for stimulation or disorientation. Disorientation will obviously be aggravated if signs within the environment are lacking or unclear.

5.12   What is the 'ABC' of dementia management?

The key to understanding problem behaviours is to obtain as much information about them as possible. This includes full details of the behaviour itself, the circumstances in which it takes place and the physical and mental state of the patient. This can be summarized as the 'ABC' of behaviour management:

■ **A**ntecedents: circumstances and precipitating factors leading to the onset of behaviour problems.
■ **B**ehaviour: description of the behaviour itself.
■ **C**onsequences: what occurs after the behaviour – how do staff, family, fellow residents and patients themselves respond to the behaviour.

In many situations, an 'ABC' analysis can allow the causes of – and possible ways of managing – problem behaviour to be identified.

5.13   How do I treat problem behaviours?

All treatment plans can be divided into three phases:

■ medical, physical or pharmacological treatments
■ psychological therapies
■ social support and assistance; environmental intervention.

The relative importance of each of these three will depend on what is being treated. In the majority of cases (at least in dementia care) a plan would be a combination of all three. It is important to note that drug treatments do not necessarily take precedence. In fact, for many situations, prescribing has a relatively limited role to play, and it can sometimes do more harm than good.

5.14   How do I treat agitation in dementia?

Agitation is an example of a 'problem' behaviour and will need to be identified and tackled but – equally importantly – understood. If the cause can be identified and removed the agitation should settle. There are many possible causes of agitation ranging from physical discomfort or pain (e.g.

constipation, blisters from ill-fitting shoes, more serious physical illness) through to depression or other emotional problems (e.g. family no longer visiting). Agitation resulting from the distress, anxiety and fear of psychotic symptoms is common. It might also be an intrinsic part of some dementia with no identifiable secondary cause.

5.15 How can a behavioural approach help a patient with agitation?

Caregivers should be encouraged to observe the episodes of agitation and record them in a systematic way (i.e. looking at the antecedents and consequences) over the course of several days. It might then be possible to identify trigger factors and attempt to eradicate or modify them. Quite often, the consequences of an episode of behavioural disturbance reinforce that behaviour, for example a shouting patient will be given more attention than a patient sitting quietly in the corner. Ways of altering the consequences of the behaviour include time out (removing the patient temporarily into a less reinforcing, positively stimulating, situation) or providing greater reinforcement of desirable behaviour (encouragement, rewards); behaviours that are not reinforced will eventually fade away (extinction). It is important that all caregivers respond in the same consistent way. Help from a community nurse or psychologist might be necessary.

5.16 What else can be done to minimize agitation?

Ensure that the patient is receiving adequate pain relief and that regular visual and hearing assessments are offered. Lighting, ambient temperature and noise levels should be satisfactory (neither too high or too low). Occupational therapy, music and relaxation techniques should be made available in residential homes or day centres. In residential homes or hospitals other disruptive patients frequently trigger agitation in others. Temporary isolation or separation from other agitated patients should be tried.

5.17 What technology is available to help keep people safe in their own home?

Straightforward and easily available devices include smoke and carbon monoxide detectors. Isolator switches for cookers and circuit breakers are available. Care line telephone systems can be installed. These allow verbal contact with an operator when an alarm cord is pulled or a button worn on a pendant is activated. The operator can then alert a preagreed carer or the emergency services.

Going one stage further is the development of devices that detect incidents such as wandering at night and falls, potentially dangerous extremes of temperature and flooding. These devices are designed to automatically alert a monitoring centre, allowing help to be organized quickly.

PATIENT QUESTIONS

5.18 It is now getting very hard to look after my father safely but I don't know whether he should move into a care home. When is the right time?

The decision to seek or recommend placement is never taken lightly and often causes significant distress and guilt in carers, who often feel that they have let their family member down. The general consensus is that patients have a right to live in their own homes if at all possible and inadequate provision of support services is not in itself a good reason for placing someone in residential care. Placement becomes necessary when a person with dementia can no longer cope safely at home, even with as much home care support as can be provided. The need for placement is likely to be triggered by behaviour resulting in fire risk, wandering (especially at night), severe neglect and repeated falls.

Patients themselves sometimes express a wish to move into residential care if they live alone and become distressed, fearful or anxious as a result of their isolation.

5.19 What can I do to stop my wife getting so agitated when I help her dress?

No one single approach works with all patients in all situations but some general advice on how to talk and deal with an agitated patient might be helpful. Try to be flexible and adapt to your wife's routine rather than expecting her to fit in with yours. If she resists help it is best to come back later rather than persist. Take into account your wife's memory or communication difficulties and any visual or hearing loss. Remember that your wife might not understand what you are trying to do for her, so speak calmly, clearly and slowly. She needs to be given adequate time to respond, both verbally and physically. Giving simple instructions one step at a time and encouraging her to perform an activity bit by bit will reduce the frustration of being unable to complete tasks.

5.20 My wife has started seeing 'small people' in our sitting room. They distress her greatly. What can I do to calm her?

These are visual hallucinations. They can be extremely vivid and life-like and your wife might be convinced that there really are strangers in your home; she might well ask if you can see them too. It is best not to 'go along' with her and say that you can. Instead, try to reassure her by gently suggesting that they are a 'trick of the mind or eyes' without getting into an argument about it. Give physical contact and try to distract her with conversation. Visual hallucinations can be caused by eye problems so it might be worth getting them checked by an optician. Neuroleptic medication (*see Qs 6.15–6.22*) can help if the hallucinations become persistent or more distressing.

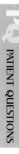

5.21 My husband has taking to pacing around the house for no apparent reason. It is wearing me down. What can I do?

There can be many causes of the agitation and restlessness that have resulted in your husband pacing. Physical discomfort or pain is one cause. Reasons could include toothache, constipation or a full bladder, all of which can be easily remedied. If your husband has recently been prescribed some new medication, check with his doctor whether this might be the cause. Make sure that he does not drink too much tea, coffee or caffeinated soft drinks.

Boredom can be a cause, particularly if he used to be a very active man. Find ways of converting his aimless wandering into more meaningful activity. Give him some small jobs around the house that he can do safely. This will make him feel more fulfilled. Go out for walks with him regularly and try to share other activities. Investigate whether there are any lunch clubs or day centres that your husband could join.

Drug treatments in dementia

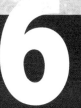

6

6.1 Are there drugs to treat dementia?

Drug treatments for dementia fall into three main categories. First, and most recent, are the drugs aimed specifically at improving, or at least slowing the decline of, cognitive function. Although these do provide useful benefits they do not offer a cure and their licensed use is currently restricted to the treatment of Alzheimer's disease.

Then there are the drugs used to treat the secondary psychiatric, psychological or behavioural symptoms or problems associated with dementia. They can be helpful but do also cause problems with adverse effects. There is currently controversy over the perceived excessive, or inappropriate use of neuroleptic drugs for patients with agitated behaviour in some residential and nursing homes, and in hospital. Last, and outside the remit of this chapter, one must consider treatment for any coexisting medical problems, many of which could be contributing to the dementia.

6.2 What drugs are available to slow cognitive decline?

Four drugs are currently available in the UK for the specific treatment of cognitive decline and associated functional impairment:

- donepezil (Aricept): a cholinesterase inhibitor
- rivastigmine (Exelon): a cholinesterase inhibitor
- galantamine (Reminyl): a cholinesterase inhibitor
- memantine (Ebixa): a glutamatergic modulator.

Currently, these are licensed only for Alzheimer's disease.

6.3 Can these drugs be used for other forms of dementia?

The drugs are licensed for Alzheimer's disease and in the UK their use is governed by national guidelines from the National Institute for Clinical Excellence (NICE; *see* Q 6.11). Despite this, there is growing evidence that the cholinesterase inhibitors can improve cognition in vascular dementia and dementia with Lewy bodies. Findings suggest that psychotic symptoms associated with dementia with Lewy bodies, as well as with Alzheimer's disease, might also improve with these drugs.

6.4 What must be considered when prescribing for patients with dementia?

It is important to consider whether the risks of prescribing a certain drug – falls, sedation, increased confusion – outweigh any possible benefits. Most patients with dementia will be elderly, with coexisting medical conditions, and taking other preparations. Reduced liver metabolism and renal excretion will prolong the drug's half life. Consequences of this include an increased risk of adverse effects. Patients with dementia are particularly vulnerable to CNS adverse effects such as sedation, movement disorders, confusion, convulsions and hallucinations. An important principle of prescribing for the elderly is, therefore, to 'start low and go slow'. That is, to commence at the lowest possible dose and to increase the dose only if necessary, according to response and the emergence of any adverse effects.

DRUG TREATMENT FOR ALZHEIMER'S DISEASE

6.5 What treatment is available for Alzheimer's disease?

Four drugs are currently licensed for the specific treatment of Alzheimer's disease: donepezil, rivastigmine and galantamine are cholinesterase inhibitors, which reversibly inhibit cholinesterase and so boost the depleted level of acetylcholine in cortical neuron systems; memantine is an NMDA receptor antagonist that modulates the activity of the excitatory neurotransmitter, glutamate, and reduces the concentration of potentially neurotoxic levels of intracellular calcium.

6.6 How useful are the cholinesterase inhibitors?

There is good evidence that, in many cases but not all, the cholinesterase inhibitors slow the rate of cognitive decline associated with progression of the disease. During the initial stages of treatment, i.e. the first 6 to 9 months, patients can show an improvement of cognitive scores compared with baseline, or their score might remain stable. Subsequently, performance might decline but scores remain higher than those estimated for untreated patients.

It is less clear to what extent effect on cognition – as measured by changes in rating scale scores of cognitive function – results in real and useful improvement in an individual's daily functioning or quality of life. However, the cholinesterase inhibitors have also been found to improve scores on tests of 'non-cognitive' parameters, such as activities of daily living and neuropsychiatric symptoms.

Longer-term outcomes might include delay in needing home care or other support services or delayed placement into residential care. This might represent a potential cost saving. It is hoped that improvements, particularly in behavioural functioning, would also lead to a lessening of carer burden. This has yet to be fully established.

6.7   How much do the cholinesterase inhibitors cost?

The drugs themselves cost around £90–£100 per month; the exact cost depends on which drug is used, the dose and any local arrangements with individual drug companies. However, 'hidden' costs will outweigh the drug costs. These include the costs of establishing and running an assessment and monitoring service, involving medical, nursing and administrative staff.

6.8   What are the side-effects of the cholinesterase inhibitors?

 All the cholinesterase inhibitors cause some gastrointestinal side-effects, including nausea and vomiting, loss of appetite and diarrhoea; headache and dizziness also occur. They should be used with caution in patients with known peptic ulcer. Other side-effects include fatigue, muscle cramps and tremor. The cholinesterase inhibitors might aggravate cardiac conduction abnormalities and it is recommended that an ECG is performed before prescribing.

Increased confusion, agitation or irritability does occur in some patients and might necessitate withdrawal of the drug. However, most adverse effects are self-limiting and dose dependent, and can be minimized by starting at a low dose and increasing the dose according to response and tolerability.

6.9   Are there any differences between the cholinesterase inhibitors currently available?

As yet, there is no evidence that one cholinesterase inhibitor is more effective than the others.

Donepezil is administered once daily compared with a twice-daily regimen for rivastigmine and galantamine. This might be an advantage for some patients or their carers. The dose of rivastigmine must be increased gradually at 4-week intervals; hence it can take longer for a patient to reach the optimal dose. A trial comparing donepezil and rivastigmine found that more patients on rivastigmine dropped out of the study because of side-effects.

All three drugs reversibly inhibit acetylcholinesterase. Rivastigmine also inhibits butryl cholinesterase and galantamine also modulates nicotinic receptors. It is not clear whether these additional actions confer significant clinical benefit.

6.10   What is the difference between memantine and the cholinesterase inhibitors?

Memantine was introduced in the UK in October 2002. So at the time of writing clinical experience of its use is limited.

The mode of action is not the same as that of the cholinesterase inhibitors (*see* Q 6.5). It is therefore possible that it could benefit patients who have not responded to the cholinesterase inhibitors. It also raises the possibility of combined therapy.

Memantine appears to confer some benefit in terms of cognitive function and functional ability in patients with moderate to severe dementia. This is in contrast to the cholinesterase inhibitors, which are licensed for patients with mild to moderate Alzheimer's disease.

6.11 Which patients should be treated with cholinesterase drugs?

In the UK, the National Institute for Clinical Excellence (NICE) has determined that all three cholinesterase inhibitors can be prescribed for patients with 'mild to moderate' Alzheimer's disease under the following conditions:

- the Alzheimer's disease must be diagnosed by a specialist
- the patient has an MMSE score >12
- only specialists (old-age psychiatrists, neurologists, care-of-the-elderly physicians) can initiate treatment
- clinicians must consider the likelihood of compliance with treatment, i.e. a carer should be available
- patients are monitored in a specialist clinic where changes to cognitive and behavioural functioning can be assessed and response to treatment ascertained.

Treatment should only be continued if, 2 to 4 months after reaching an appropriate maintenance dose, the MMSE score has improved or stayed the same and if behavioural or functional assessment shows improvement. Monitoring should take place at least every 6 months

6.12 Which patients would not be suitable for treatment with cholinesterase inhibitors?

According to the NICE guidelines, the cholinesterase inhibitors are intended for patients with Alzheimer's disease; they are not licensed for the treatment of other forms of dementia.

Prescribing of galantamine is contraindicated in severe renal impairment. Caution should be exercised in patients with cardiac conduction abnormalities, such as sick sinus syndrome, chronic obstructive airways disease and hepatic impairment. The cholinesterase inhibitors enhance the effect of suxamethonium but antagonize the effect of non-depolarizing muscle relaxants.

6.13 How long should cholinesterase inhibitor treatment be continued?

This can be anything from 4 months to 2 years or more. Evidence is emerging that the efficacy of the drugs might be sustained for as long as 5 years, although this has yet to be substantiated with placebo-controlled data.

According to NICE guidelines drugs should be continued beyond 4 months only if there is demonstrable benefit. Beyond this: 'the drug should only be continued while the patients MMSE score remains above 12 points and global, functional and behavioural condition remains at a level where the drug is having a worthwhile effect'. Clearly, there is considerable scope for interpretation and there can be no hard and fast rules.

6.14 What about gingko biloba?

Gingko biloba is an extract from the gingko tree and has traditionally been given to alleviate symptoms of 'cerebral insufficiency'. More recently, there has been some interest in its use specifically for the cognitive symptoms of dementia. Various mechanisms of action have been postulated. These include improving cerebral blood flow and having neuroprotective and antioxidant properties. Some studies have concluded that it has a beneficial effect comparable to that found with donepezil, although no double-blind trial directly comparing the two agents has so far been done.

Gingko biloba might increase bleeding times and potentiate the effect of anticoagulants. Its use should therefore be avoided in patients with clotting disorders, those taking warfarin and aspirin, and in patients awaiting surgical procedures.

6.15 What other possibilities for treatment are there?

The association between Alzheimer's pathology and the inflammatory response has led to speculation that anti-inflammatory drugs might have a protective effect. This is supported by observations that patients with arthritis or who take long-term courses of non-steroidal anti-inflammatory drugs for other reasons have a lower than expected risk of developing Alzheimer's disease. It seems less likely that these drugs will affect the progression of the disease but further research is necessary.

Estrogen increases cerebral blood flow, enhances nerve growth factor and stimulates cholinergic activity. Some epidemiological studies have found that postmenopausal women who take estrogen replacement have a reduced risk of developing Alzheimer's disease. Vitamin E and selegiline – both antioxidants – seem to show some promise. A recent double-blind, placebo-controlled trial found delayed progression of the disease in patients taking either active treatment.

The 'holy grail' of Alzheimer's drug treatment is an agent that prevents beta-amyloid deposition into plaques. Possibilities for future therapy therefore include the inhibition of the enzyme (gamma secretase) that cleaves amyloid precursor protein (APP) and forms beta-amyloid protein. Immunization with beta-amyloid protein in mice has been shown to inhibit the formation of beta-amyloid plaques and to reduce the number and density of existing plaques. The use of nerve growth factor to reverse neuronal degeneration is currently being explored and transplantation of embryonic nerve cells as has already been attempted in the treatment of Parkinson's disease.

TREATMENT OF ASSOCIATED PSYCHIATRIC AND BEHAVIOURAL SYMPTOMS

6.16 What are neuroleptic drugs?

Neuroleptic drugs (or the 'antipsychotics') include chlorpromazine, trifluoperazine and haloperidol. The newer, so-called 'atypical neuroleptics', include risperidone, clozapine, olanzapine and quetiapine (*Box 6.1*).

6.17 Why are neuroleptic drugs prescribed?

Agitation is the most common reason for prescribing neuroleptic drugs for patients with dementia, although the evidence for their efficacy, in the absence of psychosis, is relatively weak. It is important to bear in mind that this is an unlicensed indication and that the adverse effects of many of the neuroleptics include agitation and increased confusion.

6.18 How do the neuroleptics work?

The neuroleptics block dopamine receptors in the brain. Most neuroleptics also bind to cholinergic, adrenergic, histaminic and serotinergic receptors, resulting in a variety of adverse effects.

Box 6.1 Examples of the neuroleptic drugs
Conventional:
- Haloperidol
- Chlorpromazine
- Trifluoperazine
- Flupenthixol
- Promazine
- Pericyazine

Atypical:
- Amisulpiride
- Risperidone
- Olanzapine
- Quetiapine
- Clozapine

6.19 What are the main side-effects of the neuroleptics?

All the conventional neuroleptics, of which haloperidol is the most commonly prescribed, cause various movement disorders due to dopamine blockade in the nigrostriatal system.

Akathisia is persistent motor restlessness involving the upper and lower limbs. It is treated by lowering the dose of the neuroleptic.

The extrapyramidal side-effects include the parkinsonian triad of tremor, rigidity and bradykinesia. These symptoms are treated by lowering the dose or prescribing anticholinergic agents such as procyclidine.

Tardive dyskinesia is longer term and often irreversible. It is characterized by repetitive and involuntary movements of the mouth, tongue, trunk and limbs, and is often triggered by withdrawal of long-term neuroleptic medication. It is most common in older women, particularly those with a degree of cerebral damage, such as in dementia.

Other side-effects of the neuroleptics include sedation, postural hypotension and cardiac arrhythmias; antimuscarinic effects such as dry mouth, constipation, difficulty with micturition and blurred vision; endocrine changes such as galactorrhoea.

Wherever possible, the neuroleptics should be avoided in patients with dementia with Lewy bodies, who are extremely sensitive to the drugs' adverse effects. Severe parkinsonism and sedation occur.

6.20 Do neuroleptics affect cognitive function?

There is some evidence to suggest that the older neuroleptics such as chlorpromazine or thioridazine adversely affect cognitive function. A recent study of patients with dementia living at home found that the rate of cognitive decline in patients receiving neuroleptics was twice that of patients not on such medication. The patients also seemed to decline quicker following prescription compared to before. This effect is likely to be due to the anticholinergic effect of the drugs. It is less likely that haloperidol and the newer atypical neuroleptics, which have less of an anticholinergic action, will be associated with a similar decline.

6.21 What are the advantages of the newer atypical neuroleptics?

The atypical neuroleptics are more selective. Consequently, they cause fewer movement disorder effects such as parkinsonism. They have a lower anticholinergic activity and also cause less sedation. They therefore have less of an impact both on the patient's cognitive function and on mobility.

6.22 What are the disadvantages of the atypical neuroleptics?

The main one is cost. The atypical neuroleptics, dose for dose, cost between three and five times that of haloperidol. Although in general they are much better tolerated, they are not without adverse effects. At doses above 3 mg daily, risperidone causes extrapyramidal symptoms in older patients with dementia. Other side-effects include dizziness and postural hypotension. There have been some recent reports of an increased risk of cerebrovascular events in patients taking Risperidone. The clinical implications of this are, at the time of writing, unclear.

6.23 What do you recommend I prescribe?

Neuroleptic drugs should not be prescribed without having first attempted to identify and resolve the cause of the agitation. Alternative non-drug treatment options should also have been considered.

Risperidone 0.5–1.0 mg daily has been found to be effective compared with placebo in reducing psychosis and behavioural disturbance in hospitalized patients with dementia. Olanzapine 2.5–10 mg daily seems similarly effective but might be more sedating and can cause weight gain and hyperglycaemia. Quetiapine is another atypical neuroleptic that is well tolerated in this patient group.

6.24 What other drugs are used for agitation?

Antidepressants or anxiolytics should be used if the agitation is a consequence of a depressive episode or anxiety. The so-called mood stabilizers – carbamazepine or valproate – can be tried for agitation associated with lability of mood. Low doses of a benzodiazepine might also be considered where a neuroleptic has been ineffective or the adverse effects are unacceptable. Lorazepam 0.5 mg once or twice daily might be effective.

6.25 Which antidepressants are used in patients with dementia?

Depression in patients with dementia is not uncommon. It usually responds to conventional antidepressant medication. However, coexisting cerebral disease is associated with a poorer outcome in terms of speed or completeness of recovery. It is important to remind the patient and carer that any antidepressant will take 2 weeks to start to work and response thereafter will be progressive over the ensuing 2–3 months. The principle of starting at low doses applies. The minimum effective dose should be used.

The two most commonly prescribed classes of antidepressant are the tricyclic and related antidepressants and the selective serotonin reuptake inhibitors (SSRIs). Other classes include the monoamine oxidase inhibitors (e.g. phenelzine) and the serotonin and noradrenaline reuptake inhibitor (SNRI) venlafaxine (*Box 6.2*).

6.26 How do the tricyclic antidepressants work?

Tricyclic antidepressants (TCAs) inhibit the reuptake of monoamines in the synaptic cleft, thus increasing the available supply of monoamine

> **Box 6.2 Some examples of antidepressant medication**
> **Selective serotonin inhibitors (SSRIs):**
> - Fluoxetine
> - Paroxetine
> - Citalopram
> - Sertraline
>
> **Serotonin and noradrenaline reuptake inhibitor:**
> - Venlafaxine
>
> **Tricyclic and related antidepressants:**
> - Amitriptyline
> - Dothiepin
> - Lofepramine
> - Imipramine
> - Trazodone
>
> **Monoamine oxidase inhibitors (MAOIs):**
> - Phenelzine
> - Moclobamide
> - Tranylcypromine

neurotransmitters to the postsynaptic receptors. They also block the uptake of the monoamines: serotonin, dopamine and noradrenaline, and have antihistaminic, anticholinergic and adrenergic effects.

6.27 What are the main adverse effects of the TCAs?

 Adverse effects vary across individual drugs in this group but include dry mouth sedation, blurred vision, constipation and exacerbation of prostatism. They can precipitate cardiac arrythmias and lower seizure threshold. The latter might be important in a patient with dementia who is at increased risk of epileptic seizures. The TCAs are potentially fatal in overdose.

6.28 Should TCAs be prescribed for depressed patients with dementia?

 TCAs should not be the first choice of treatment for depressed patients with dementia.

Older people are more likely to have glaucoma or urinary outflow problems, which might be aggravated by tricyclics. The anticholinergic effect can worsen the patients' cognitive function or trigger delirium or neuropsychiatric symptoms such as hallucinations. The TCAs with the greatest anticholinergic activity are imipramine and amitriptyline, which should therefore be avoided; lofepramine and nortriptyline have lower anticholinergic activity. Trazodone is commonly used in patients with agitation because it is mildly sedating and relatively free of anticholinergic activity, so minimizing impairment of cognitive function.

Sedation is likely to be a problem and the potential consequences of an accidental (or deliberate) overdose by an unsupervised older person are serious. The more sedative tricyclics are amitriptyline, trimipramine and dothiepin.

6.29 What about the SSRIs?

 The SSRIs are the antidepressants of choice in older patients. On the whole, they are much better tolerated than the other classes of antidepressants but they are not without their adverse effects. These include loss of appetite, nausea and abdominal pain. This can be problematic for older patients who have already lost weight as a result of dementia and depression. They are relatively safe in overdose.

6.30 What other unwanted effects are associated with the SSRIs?

 A withdrawal syndrome has been associated with SSRIs with a short half-life, such as paroxetine. Symptoms include agitation, tremor, headache and anxiety. It is necessary to reinstate the SSRI but to consider switching to a longer half-life drug, e.g. fluoxetine, and then to withdraw the drug slowly by reducing the dose gradually over 4 weeks.

Hyponatraemia due to inappropriate secretion of antidiuretic hormone is an occasional and usually incidental finding in patients on SSRIs, although it is also associated with other classes of antidepressant. It is more common in older people and its clinical significance is uncertain, although reduced plasma sodium can cause cerebral effects such as increased confusion, convulsions and drowsiness.

6.31 What should I do if a patient develops hyponatraemia?

Withdraw the antidepressant and monitor the serum sodium regularly. Switch to an antidepressant of a different class, starting at a low dose and increasing the dose slowly, while continuing to monitor the sodium. Seek specialist advice if the serum sodium is below 125 mmol/L.

 PATIENT QUESTIONS

6.32 Is medication for dementia addictive?

There is no evidence that the drugs currently licensed for the treatment of Alzheimer's disease are addictive. It is possible that a more rapid deterioration of the condition is noticed when the drug is discontinued, most likely after a prolonged course of treatment. If this does occur, going back on treatment can temporarily improve the situation.

Other drugs that can be given to a patient with dementia include antidepressants and tranquilizers of various kinds. Some antidepressants have been linked to unpleasant 'withdrawal' effects, including nervousness and agitation. Sedatives such as diazepam might also cause increased anxiety when discontinued. Seek medical advice before attempting to stop such medication and always cut down the dose gradually rather than stopping suddenly.

6.33　Will there ever be a cure for Alzheimer's disease?

The drugs that are currently available act on the symptoms of Alzheimer's disease and not the disease itself. Unfortunately, at the time of writing, there are no drugs 'in the pipeline' that will repair the damage to the brain that Alzheimer's disease has caused. However, much work has been done – and continues to be done – to find out exactly why and how these brain changes occur, and who is most at risk of developing the disease. There is, therefore, much hope that a treatment will be developed to prevent the disease taking a hold in the first place.

6.34　I would prefer not to take chemical preparations, are there any herbal remedies available?

Gingko biloba is readily available over the counter at pharmacies or by mail order; some reports suggest that it might improve memory but this is uncertain and there is no strong evidence for it being effective against Alzheimer's disease. Although it is relatively safe it can react with some types of medication, such as warfarin. So if you are thinking about taking it, always check with your doctor first.

Sage has been used since ancient times to aid failing memory. It has antioxidant properties and has also been found to have a cholinesterase effect along similar lines to the drugs described above.

6.35　Are there any homeopathic or other complementary therapies available for dementia?

A few common homeopathic remedies claim to help 'dullness of mind', 'vagueness' 'stupefaction' and other dementia-related symptoms. Evidence of the effectiveness of these remedies is lacking.

The role of nutritional supplements, including vitamins, minerals and essential fatty acids, in the prevention of dementia is arousing much interest at the moment. There is some – but by no means conclusive – evidence to suggest that the antioxidant vitamins E and C, and omega 3 fatty acids (in fish oil) might have a protective effect.

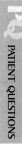

PQ PATIENT QUESTIONS

Services for people with dementia

7

7.1   What kinds of services are available for people with dementia?

An important principle underpinning services for people with dementia in the UK is its multidisciplinary and multiagency nature. Primary healthcare services remain central to patient care, with secondary specialist services providing input where necessary. Specialist psychiatric or psychological evaluation and treatment, community monitoring and support, occupational therapy assessment and rehabilitation can all be accessed. Teams comprising professionals from a range of healthcare disciplines, and local authority social services, are supported by voluntary agencies. Relevant and timely treatment and support is intended to maximize patients' independence and safety, allowing them to remain at home for as long as possible.

Two groups of patients with dementia are less well provided for. Younger patients with dementia have specific needs, which are not being properly met by existing services, and patients from different racial groups also have specific needs. In a multiethnic society it has become increasingly important to take into account language and cultural aspects when planning and delivering health and social care.

The answers to the following questions are written from a UK perspective; the general principles apply more broadly.

PSYCHIATRIC SERVICES

7.2   When should I refer to an old-age psychiatrist?

The introduction of drugs for Alzheimer's disease has led to a demand for patients to be seen by specialist old-age psychiatry services in the early stages of their condition. Hitherto, patients were often looked after by their GP while their condition progressed and referred only at the point of crisis because of behavioural disturbance and carer stress. At this point, urgent admission to hospital was often the only option. Diagnosing the condition and evaluating the situation at an earlier stage allows a management plan to be established, including monitoring the progress of the condition and providing advice and support to patient and carer, as well as perhaps implementing treatment. This itself might avert a crisis but it also means that if one does occur then fully informed decisions can be made.

Not all patients with dementia need to be referred to an old-age psychiatrist, and not all services can cope with the increased workload that early referral brings. It is also true that the standards of specialist dementia care services vary across the country. For these reasons, referral guidelines or pathways are being established. Generally, referral should be considered if any of the following apply:

- there is doubt over diagnosis
- the patient is being considered for treatment with acetylcholinesterase inhibitors
- there is significant impairment of daily functioning
- there is evidence of carer stress
- the patient's behaviour is dangerous
- there are associated psychiatric symptomatology or behavioural problem.

In addition, many social services request an old-age psychiatrists' opinion when considering in which residential home a patient would best be placed.

7.3 Do old-age psychiatrists see younger adults with dementia?

Some do and some don't. Specific funded services for younger adults with dementia are rare but many old-age psychiatry services offer at least an assessment service for this group of patients. However, younger patients with dementia are currently ill served in day-hospital or ward facilities designed for a much older patient group.

7.4 When should I refer to a neurologist?

There can be no hard and fast rules because services differ across the country. Some neurologists are more interested in dementia than others. Most neurologists, particularly in district general hospitals, also have long waiting lists! Referral might also depend on whether the local psychiatric service provides a good dementia assessment service for younger as well as older patients; not all of them do.

In general, patients with one or more of the following features should be referred to a neurologist:

- onset under the age of 65 years especially if there is a strong family history of dementia
- rapid progression of dementia
- neurological symptoms and signs, such as myoclonic jerks, ataxia, personality, seizures or behavioural change
- abnormal neurological signs on examination.

7.5 What are National Service Frameworks?

National Service Frameworks (NSF) are intended to improve standards of care and to reduce variations in health and social services across the UK. They are sets of national standards of health and social care drawn up by the Department of Health (UK).

7.6 What does the NSF have to do with dementia?

The most recent NSF to be published was the National Service Framework for Older People. This requires services to ensure – amongst many other things – that patients with suspected dementia receive a prompt diagnosis, that there is easy access to specialist care and appropriate treatments, and that carers receive the advice and support they need.

7.7 According to the NSF, what is the role of the GP?

It is expected that specialist services will offer training to those working in primary care on diagnosis and treatment of dementia. They will work together to draw up agreed protocols for the identification and appropriate referral of patients; this is likely to involve the use of rating scales. GPs will also be required to provide closer monitoring of patients in residential care who are receiving psychotropic medication.

THE MULTIDISCIPLINARY TEAM

7.8 What is a community psychiatric nurse?

A community psychiatric nurse (CPN) is a trained mental health nurse. Usually working within a community mental health team, the CPN plays an important role in coordinating the care that a patient receives from the specialist service. The CPN is involved in the assessment and ongoing monitoring of patients with dementia in the community; both in their homes and in residential homes. The CPN acts as an advocate for the patient and the carer, liaising on their behalf with primary and specialist care services, as well as other agencies, to ensure that appropriate help is given. CPNs are often involved in running lunch clubs, support groups for patient and spouses, and, in residential care settings, are also a valuable source of advice and support to care staff. Many CPNs are associated with specific GP practices and might take referrals for assessment in their own right. They are well placed to advise and educate GPs and other primary care colleagues on dementia assessment and care.

7.9 What does an occupational therapist do?

Occupational therapy is the treatment of physical and psychiatric conditions through specific activities in order to help people reach their maximum level of function in all aspects of daily life. Occupational therapists, working within the multidisciplinary team, are involved in both the assessment and treatment of patients with dementia. Assessment of a patient's ability to perform activities of daily living – ideally at home – is a crucial element of discharge planning. Such an assessment will influence the decision as to whether a patient can live safely at home, the type of home care to be arranged and the need for any adaptations to the home.

An occupational therapist might be involved in the treatment of a patient in a number of ways. These include advising a patient of techniques to overcome memory loss, or exercises intended to preserve existing functional ability. Activities designed to increase social interaction and to enhance communication or sensory stimulation are also employed.

7.10 What does a psychologist do?

Psychologists working with patients with dementia perform several functions. Psychometric assessment is the objective measurement of a patient's cognitive function; and an assessment using a series of neuropsychological tests helps in dementia screening and the differential diagnosis of patients with dementia.

Psychologists are also instrumental in coordinating and supervising the various psychological treatments, and behavioural management, of patients with dementia. As such they work closely with nursing and occupational therapy staff on wards and in day hospitals.

7.11 What is a memory clinic?

The function of a memory clinic is to provide a comprehensive evaluation of a patient's cognitive impairment at one, or at most, two clinic visits. There is no standardized model and memory clinics vary widely; indeed, not all districts have them. Most offer an assessment by a psychiatrist and either a neurologist or a physician. Psychometric testing by a psychologist is desirable. Nurses and occupational therapists might also be involved. Some clinics have the facilities for CT, MRI or functional imaging.

Most memory clinics see patients referred by GPs or hospital doctors, although some accept self-referrals. The advantages of a memory clinic are the ease of access to a comprehensive assessment and the potential benefits of early detection of a dementing condition. However, only a small proportion of patients can be seen in such a clinic. Patients referred to such clinics tend to be younger and have unusual symptoms or an atypical presentation. Experience has shown that a significant proportion of patients seen have apparent cognitive impairment secondary to an affective disorder.

A further development of the memory clinic aims to provide a 'one-stop shop' for all people with dementia irrespective of age. Here a patient can be assessed and receive information about their condition and advice about benefits and support services all under one roof.

DAY SERVICES

7.12 What happens in a day hospital?

Day hospitals are organized by health services, often within the same premises as inpatient and outpatient facilities. Day hospitals act as a 'buffer' between the wards and the community. Patients can be admitted to a day hospital in preference to a ward to minimize the disorientating and deskilling effect of completely removing someone from a familiar environment. Attendance at day hospital might also smooth the transition between hospital and home following discharge.

Day hospitals are staffed by nurses, occupational therapists and physiotherapists – usually with support from medical staff and psychologists. Patients might be admitted to a day hospital for continuing assessment of cognition, behaviour and activities of daily living. Treatment in day hospitals takes place in groups, as well as on an individual basis, and might include enhancement of social functioning, coping with bereavement and anxiety management.

Another important function of a day hospital is to provide respite for carers by looking after a patient for one or two days per week. Staff at the day hospital are a useful point of contact and source of advice for carers.

7.13 What is the difference between a day centre and a day hospital?

Day centres are funded, managed and run by local authorities and/or voluntary agencies, such as Age Concern. They are run by care staff who do not have medical or nurse training; there is usually little or no input from doctors, although many old age psychiatry services provide some form of outreach and liaison with local day centres. Day centres are primarily concerned with social contact and stimulation, as well as providing respite for carers. Generally, the main functions of day hospitals – as far as dementia care is concerned – are assessment, monitoring and treatment. Day hospitals are free. Most day centres charge, at least for the meals provided and the transport.

SOCIAL AND COMMUNITY SERVICES

7.14 What role does a social worker play in dementia care?

Social workers are based in various settings: in general hospitals, as part of a specialist mental health team and in the community. They assess a patient's need for community care services such as home help, meals on wheels and day care. Decisions about type of care required, or whether placement into a home is necessary, are based on assessments of both need and risk, usually in consultation with other members of the specialist or primary care team. Social workers are then responsible for arranging such care through separate, usually private, agencies, and monitoring its acceptance and effectiveness. The social worker assists patients and their families to choose appropriate residential homes and advises about benefits that might be available. Inevitably, social workers also play an important role in counselling patients and carers.

7.15 What is an approved social worker?

Approved social workers have undergone specific training in the use of the mental health act. Their assessment and subsequent 'application', along with that of two doctors who make 'medical recommendations', is necessary when admitting a patient under the mental health act.

7.16 How can a home carer help someone with dementia?

Home-careworkers are arranged through social services but normally provided by private agencies; they perform essential domestic tasks. These include, where necessary, helping with dressing, washing and shaving. Home-careworkers might also do shopping, prepare meals and remind the patient to take medication. They can, therefore, help maintain a person, who is unable to manage independently, at home. Home-careworkers might be the only regular human contact for an isolated patient and are therefore in a good position to alert other services if problems arise.

7.17 What is 'respite care'?

Admitting a patient with dementia for a short period into hospital or a residential home can give valuable respite to a carer. Many carers find respite care the most valuable form of support, especially if it can be provided at very short notice. Availability varies across the UK and can be provided via social services or through the local old age psychiatry service or both. In the case of hospital provision, this is usually for patients who cannot be properly managed elsewhere. Respite in hospital also provides the opportunity for regular reviews of mental state and physical condition. Carers occasionally worry that frequent periods of respite care might worsen a patient's disorientation and it is not unusual for a patient to become more agitated for a while on returning home. Clearly, each case has to be taken on its merits. If respite care significantly worsens the situation at home it might be better not to persevere with it.

7.18 What is 'continuing care'?

'Continuing care' refers to the provision of longer-term hospital care for patients who, it is agreed, cannot be managed properly in any other setting, e.g. private or local authority residential or nursing homes. Such patients usually have severe or difficult-to-manage forms of behavioural disturbance. A decision to provide continuing care is reviewed regularly and should involve next of kin and other family members.

7.19 What is an 'EMI home'?

'EMI' stands for 'elderly mentally infirm' and is one category of residential or nursing home. It indicates that such a home employs sufficient numbers of staff who have received relevant training to manage patients with dementia.

7.20 What other community care services are there?

There are other kinds of community-based service. Many are organized through voluntary agencies and charities rather than the statutory health or social services. Not all are available everywhere:

- lunch clubs
- sitting services, whereby a volunteer looks after a dementia sufferer in their own home for 2 to 3 hours while the carer goes out
- meals on wheels: this often involves delivering a week's worth of frozen ready meals, which the carer or home help heats up when required
- laundry services and/or provision of pads for someone who is incontinent
- chiropody, district nurse (arranged through the GP).

7.21 What is an Admiral nurse?

In a number of areas of the UK, specialist mental health nurses work solely for and with carers of patients with dementia. These posts are joint initiatives with health trusts and the Dementia Relief Trust. Admiral nurses aim to provide information and practical and emotional support to carers of all ages. An important aspect of their work is helping a carer who is considering placing a relative in residential care. Recognizing that this decision is frequently traumatic for the relative, supportive contact is often maintained afterwards. Admiral Nurses liaise with other agencies to ensure that appropriate services are implemented at the right time and are also involved in training of other professionals in dementia care.

7.22 What is the Alzheimer's society?

Previously known as the Alzheimer's Disease Society, the Alzheimer's Society is a charitable organization dedicated to improving the quality of life for people with dementia and their carers. The Society does this in a number of ways. It supplies information in the form of newsletters and advice leaflets to carers, and provides reports and opinion on aspects of dementia and dementia care to government and to the media. The Alzheimer's Society funds a very active research programme.

Through its local branches, the Society facilitates self-help and carer support groups. These allow carers to meet others in a similar situation to share information and advice on dealing with practical problems, or with coping with the stress of caring. Local Alzheimer's Society branches might also fund respite care and sitting services.

YOUNGER PEOPLE WITH DEMENTIA

7.23 What is the prevalence of dementia in younger people?

It has been estimated that the prevalence of dementia in the 45- to 65-year-old age range is approximately 50 per 100 000, with the overall number of younger people with dementia in the UK being just under 20 000.

7.24 What are the causes of dementia in younger people?

Younger people do develop Alzheimer's disease but this, relatively, accounts for a smaller proportion of cases than in older people. Frontotemporal dementia, vascular dementia and alcohol-related dementia are other important causes. Dementia associated with Aids and Huntington's disease will also account for a number of cases.

7.25 Are there any particular problems with diagnosis in this age group?

First, the spectrum of diagnoses is different than that in older people. Unfamiliar clinical presentations of unfamiliar disorders, such as subtle changes in personality or behaviour in frontotemporal dementia, will lead to a delay in recognizing and diagnosing the problem. One recent study found a mean time to diagnosis of over 3 years. Even in specialist clinics accurate diagnosis might not be possible in the early stages.

Second, there is no consensus over which specialist service should be responsible for such patients. The GP therefore might not know who to refer to: neurologists, general psychiatrists or old-age psychiatrists. This risks delaying diagnosis further.

7.26 What other implications are there for younger people with dementia?

There might well be dependent children still living at home. Children are likely to suffer psychological and emotional problems as a consequence of having a parent with dementia. Conflict with the parent, who might have become emotionally detached, irritable or disinhibited, as well as difficulties at school have been reported.

Financial problems as a result of loss of employment or forced early retirement through ill health are common. In many cases, financial commitments remain in the form of mortgages, loans, school fees and so on. There is then pressure for a spouse to seek or remain at work, while at the same time having to deal with the competing demands and responsibility of looking after children as well as the patient.

Patients with early-onset dementia are likely to have a high prevalence of psychiatric and behavioural disorders. For example, in one study 49% were depressed and around 30% were anxious and/or aggressive. These factors will lead to greater strain in carers and an increased demand on support services.

7.27 What services are available for younger people with dementia?

There are few funded, specialized services for this group of patients. Facilities for the care of dementia – wards, day hospitals, day centres – have usually been designed and are run with older people in mind. But activities that are suitable for an 85-year-old woman with Alzheimer's disease are unlikely to be appropriate for a 50-year-old man with frontal lobe dementia. Therefore younger people with dementia find themselves effectively excluded from facilities such as day centres.

Relatively few patients and their carers are in regular contact with a social worker. In hospital, patients must share wards with either younger patients with functional psychiatric disorders such as schizophrenia, or with older patients with dementia. Neither is satisfactory for several reasons. A general psychiatry unit is unlikely to have the skills and resources to cope with the needs of someone with significant cognitive impairment. Old-age psychiatry units, although experienced in managing the condition, are not well suited to caring for physically robust younger patients.

DEMENTIA IN PATIENTS FROM DIFFERENT ETHNIC GROUPS

7.28 Does the prevalence of dementia differ amongst ethnic groups?

The prevalence of dementia in different ethnic groups or populations is not well documented, but a number of trends are emerging. Studies from the US have found a higher incidence of dementias in African–American and Hispanic people than in whites. Higher rates of dementia have been found in African–Caribbeans in the UK compared with white residents. Physical conditions that increase the risk of cognitive decline – and in particular cerebrovascular disease, hypertension, diabetes and stroke – are all more prevalent in African–Caribbean populations.

7.29 What are the problems with diagnosing dementia in non-white ethnic populations?

There are certain barriers that inhibit an individual from seeking any form of health care. These include cultural beliefs about illness, language and, in many countries, economic barriers. Regarding dementia specifically, the assessment of the condition is hampered by the inadequacy of commonly used screening instruments, which were developed for white populations. Most screening tests will underestimate the cognitive function of an individual whose first language is not English, who belongs to a non-white culture and who has had less formal education.

7.30 Do the associated symptoms of dementia differ amongst ethnic groups?

Various studies have indicated that the rates of depression and anxiety are lower in African–Caribbean patients with dementia than in white patients. Rates of psychosis might be higher.

7.31 Should a patient's ethnic group be taken into account when assessing dementia?

Because of language and cultural differences, existing cognitive tests validated in Western populations might not accurately measure the extent of cognitive impairment. Language barriers cannot always be overcome. The use of translators, especially English-speaking family members, is associated with diagnostic error and inaccurate assessment of level of cognitive function. Work is being done to adapt and validate the MMSE for different ethnic groups. In the meantime, a simple test has been proposed as a basic, general screen for dementia where language barriers exist. This comprises a three-item recall test and the clock-drawing test.

7.32 Should a patient's ethnic group be taken into account when managing dementia?

Patients with dementia from non-white backgrounds are more likely to rely on family members for their care, and for longer. These family members will need counselling, information on dementia and help in caring that is sensitive to their particular needs. Acceptance of community-based support and residential care by patients from ethnic minorities is less widespread. This can partly be explained by cultural norms emphasizing the important role of the extended family. But it also reflects the relative lack of provision of culturally specific care services.

GPs working in areas with large ethnic minority populations need to respond to the needs of patients with dementia and their carers within these communities. Recruiting staff from the local area, training others on cultural issues, providing information leaflets in appropriate languages can all help to inform the local population about dementia and the facilities that are available to help them.

Problems faced by carers and their families

8

CARERS AND CARER STRESS

8.1 Who are the carers?

Dementia does not just affect the individual sufferer. The cognitive decline, impairment of ability, behavioural change and psychiatric symptoms all take their toll on spouses and everyone else who is involved in the person's wellbeing. Health and social services can provide only limited assistance with the day-to-day care of a person with dementia. Families, friends and neighbours remain the most important sources of support and the care of these informal and unpaid carers is a vital aspect of dementia management.

Relatives who care are predominantly female. Male carers are usually the husbands of women with dementia. The main or only carer for around 50% of patients with dementia is someone of a similar age – a spouse or sibling. These people are therefore probably elderly and perhaps also in need of care in their own right.

8.2 What is 'carer stress'?

Carer stress is a consequence of caring for an individual. It is influenced by the nature of the care burden itself – the physical and emotional demands on the carer – and variables within the carer, such as coping skills and strategies. Other factors include availability of support networks and services for both carer and patient, demands on carer's financial resources and any additional demands on the carer's time and energy, such as child care.

8.3 What causes stress in carers?

Studies suggest that it is not necessarily the severity of a sufferer's cognitive impairment that predicts stress or strain in carers. Functional impairment of activities of daily living or of self-care is also clearly important, as this will dictate the amount and nature of practical help required. But the behaviour of the individual being cared for seems to have the biggest impact. This need not be extreme. Repetitive questioning, constant demands or loss of initiative that requires frequent prompting can be very stressful over the course of months or years. Restlessness, agitation, argumentativeness or aggression quickly become both an emotional and physical strain. This is compounded if there are communication difficulties, which tend to occur secondarily to dementia-induced language impairment but might also be the result of hearing loss with reluctance to use a hearing aid. Loss of visual acuity also affects dementia patients and their carers.

Stress will be exacerbated by social isolation. Carer often have little time for themselves. They might have to give up work (with consequent financial implications), hobbies or other social pursuits. Friends often become increasingly reluctant to visit. They might feel uncomfortable or embarrassed, particularly if the sufferer has become disinhibited.

The causes of stress amongst carers can be summarized as follows:

- practical: the physical demands of providing practical help
- behavioural: problems such as agitation, incontinence and aggression causing distress, fear, anxiety and lack of sleep
- interpersonal: sadness over the 'loss' of a spouse, tension and arguments
- social: loss of contact with friends, being 'tied' to the house.

8.4   Which carers are most likely to experience stress?

The following characteristics predict an increased risk of carer stress:

- previous tendency to suffer stress and a history of depression or anxiety
- inflexible approach to routine
- excessive fastidiousness in respect to personal hygiene and household cleanliness
- where the carer is a spouse, an unsatisfactory marital relationship; recent marriages are more at risk than long-standing ones
- a reluctance to seek help from outside sources
- lack of support, i.e. few friends, confidantes, etc.
- lack of information about the condition/behaviour, etc.

8.5   What are the consequences of carer stress?

Carers run a higher risk of developing depression and anxiety. In one study, the prevalence of depression in carers seeking help was found to be 26%. Carers are also more likely to become physically ill, or to rate themselves as sick.

Stress or resulting psychiatric morbidity is likely to affect the care provided in a number of ways. Carers might detach themselves from the emotional aspect of caring, doing the necessary practical tasks in a distant, automatic manner. They might decide that they cannot cope any longer, triggering a crisis requiring emergency placement or hospitalization. Psychological morbidity, family conflict and financial problems are all – not surprisingly – associated with earlier placement into care.

Unfortunately, a further consequence of carer stress is the risk of abuse of the patient; both physical and emotional (*see Qs 8.9–8.18*).

COPING WITH STRESS

8.6   What coping styles are there?

There are various coping styles and techniques, some of which are more adaptive and useful to the changing demands of the caregiving situation than others.

One model of coping strategy outlines the differences between behavioural (or problem-focused) and psychological (or emotional) responses. In the behavioural coping response, carers take a relatively dispassionate view of the tasks in hand, to organize and prioritize and, crucially, to seek out help and information from other sources. The psychological coping response involves efforts to make sense of the stressful experience in a variety of ways. Another model emphasizes the distinction between 'care managing' – whereby carers coordinate and manage care provided by other agencies – and 'care providing' – in which the carers actually perform most of the caring tasks. Males are more likely to be care managers whereas females are more often care providers.

A further dimension is the degree of emotional and geographical closeness achieved by carers. 'Distancing' involves not visiting and introducing help from other sources or, alternatively, continuing to provide practical care but detaching emotionally from the situation. By contrast, 'enmeshment' results in carer and patient becoming emotionally dependent on each other to the extent that offers of help from others are perceived as a threat.

8.7 What is successful coping?

Carers who can remain flexible to the changing demands of the situation and are willing to seek help, advice and information are more likely to cope. Adopting problem-focused strategies and taking a step back from the often overwhelming emotions of a caring situation are also likely reduce the risk of stress.

Coping techniques that are likely to be counterproductive or harmful include:

- those involving blame (blaming the person not the illness or blaming oneself as a carer for the situation)
- excessive control or coercion
- denial of the extent of the problem.

8.8 What can be done to lessen carer stress?

Assistance to carers takes various forms (see Chapter 7). There is good evidence that appropriate support can improve psychological morbidity in carers. However, to be effective it should be commenced early and provided consistently. Probably the most important are the provision of respite and day care, and the availability of support groups.

Support groups can provide a setting where advice or training can be given in caring or coping techniques, perhaps by more experienced carers. The provision of relevant factual information and the knowledge that professional support can be provided promptly when necessary is invaluable.

ELDER ABUSE

8.9 What is 'elder abuse'?

Elder abuse has been defined as 'a repeated act against, or failure to act for, an elderly person, which causes distress or damage, and so prevents the living of a full life'.

It is therefore wide ranging and includes more than assault, sexual and verbal abuse and deliberate physical neglect; financial exploitation and emotional neglect are also examples of elder abuse. It includes omission of care, which can be due to lack of awareness or passive acceptance, as well as deliberate neglect. All who work with older people should be alert to its possibility and be aware of local reporting mechanisms and protocols.

8.10 Where does elder abuse occur?

Elder abuse occurs in all settings, including hospitals and residential homes, as well as in individuals' homes.

8.11 How common is elder abuse?

A number of population surveys have been done both in Europe and North America, which indicate a prevalence of around 4% of older people being subject to a form of abuse at any one time. Prevalence is likely to be much higher for at-risk groups (see below). Abuse committed by carers and other family members in a patient's own home might not ever come to light; abuse occurring in residential homes and hospital wards is more likely to be witnessed. One study reported that one-fifth of care-home staff had seen another staff member physically abuse a resident. A recent questionnaire study carried out by the Social Services Inspectorate found that 50% of GPs surveyed had come across an example of elder abuse within the past year.

8.12 What are the problems with its detection?

Elder abuse can remain undetected for a number of reasons. The older person might not recognize the abuse or neglect for what it is, or might not report it because of difficulties with communication, not being able to access an appropriate confidante or not knowing who to talk to about it. A person is unlikely to divulge the abuse if the abusing carer is always present at appointments.

The abused older person often feels stigmatized and might fear reprisals. Anxiety about being 'put in a home' can inhibit complaints about quality of care. Older people might also think that nobody would believe them ('it's my word against his'). Signs of abuse might not be evident when the patient is fully clothed in a clinic or day centre and evidence of injury might be inconclusive. It is important to remember that thin, elderly skin tears easily and that old, osteoporotic bones are prone to fracture.

8.13 What are the predisposing factors leading to abuse?

Certain factors within the carer (*Box 8.1*), the person receiving care (*Box 8.2*) and the environment in which care takes place (*Box 8.3*) make the likelihood of elder abuse more likely.

Box 8.1 Carers: factors raising the likelihood of abuse
- Inadequate support in their caring role
- Increased stress on other aspects of their life
- Financial dependency on the individual receiving care
- Poor communication between carer and patient
- History of family violence
- Alcohol or substance misuse

Box 8.2 Patients: factors that can predict abuse
- Female
- Cognitive impairment: patients with dementia are twice as likely to suffer from physical abuse as someone who does not have dementia
- Impairment of physical ability
- History of falls and minor injuries (described by the carer as 'accident prone')
- Living with an adult offspring
- Socially isolated but dependent on others
- Verbally abusive towards carers or otherwise showing challenging behaviour

Box 8.3 The caring environment: factors predisposing to elder abuse
- Cramped or substandard living conditions
- Social isolation
- When the institution in which the individual lives has a history of providing substandard care

8.14 Which residential homes are most likely to be associated with abuse?

Homes with a high turnover of young, untrained and inexperienced staff are most likely to have problems with abuse. Abuse is more likely to occur when staff are unsupervised or working in isolation. Specialist homes that offer a range of diversional activities for their clients and which have a high staff:patient ratio are less associated with abuse.

8.15 How can possible abuse be identified?

Various screening tests have been developed but none is yet in regular use in the UK. It is important to be alert to the possibility of abuse and to be aware of risk factors (*see Q 8.13*). Indicators of possible abuse include signs of injury that are suggestive of abuse, for example burns, multiple bruising and genital injury, particularly when there has been delay in seeking medical help or where explanations are inconsistent. More subtle signs of physical neglect are poor personal hygiene and malnutrition. Appearing fearful or withdrawn in the presence of a carer might be a warning sign. Being low in mood or anxious in the home but more content in another setting, e.g. day centre should also initiate enquiry

8.16 What screening questions could I ask to check for abuse?

- Do you need help in looking after yourself?
- Do you know anyone you can turn to in a crisis?
- Do you have enough privacy?
- Can you describe for me a typical day?
- Are you uncomfortable with anyone in your family?
- Have you suffered any injuries recently? Describe them.
- Who makes important decisions about your life?
- Does your carer drink too much?

8.17 What should I do if I suspect abuse?

Having identified an instance of suspected abuse, further enquiry must be undertaken. This will require detailed interviews with the patient, carer and other informants. In the case of suspected abuse in a residential home, the situation should be discussed with the manager, the Social Services department and possibly also with the local authority responsible for registering the home.

The exact procedure to be followed will depend on the form of abuse, the immediate risk to the patient and the setting in which the abuse has occurred. Urgent admission to hospital, placement into residential care or moving to another home might be necessary. The

> Police should be involved at an early stage if there is good evidence of serious assault or theft.
>
> Lesser degrees of abuse require a more considered approach to avoid distressing the victim further but also to maintain the support of the carer involved. Most local authorities and elderly mental health services in the UK will have a procedure for managing cases of suspected abuse that will involve alerting, reporting, investigating and monitoring the problem. Social workers and community nurses often take the lead role, in many cases with the Adult Protection Unit of the local Police force providing support.

8.18 What questions could I ask when interviewing a suspected victim of abuse?

The following questions can help confirm whether abuse is taking place. Clearly, follow-up questions will be needed to gain more details. Answers need to be interpreted according to the patient's cognitive function and language skills. Non-verbal responses to some questions might be as meaningful as a spoken response.

- Has anyone tried to hurt you?
- Have you been forced to do things you did not want to do?
- Has anyone tried to threaten you with going into a home?
- Has anyone taken things from you without permission?
- Has anyone confined you in a room or at home without your permission?
- Has anyone refused to provide you with food or medication?
- Has anyone made you sign a document that you did not understand?
- Are you afraid of anyone?

PQ PATIENT QUESTIONS

8.19 Is it common to feel guilty about considering residential care for my relative?

Guilt is extremely common. Many carers worry that considering placement into residential care is a betrayal of their loved one. They might have promised never to relinquish care, or be concerned about the quality of care that a home would provide. They might see it as a sign of failure – of having given up. However, it is important to recognize that caring for someone with dementia can be a heavy burden, both physically and emotionally, and that everyone has their limits. Some patients just cannot be looked after safely in the home, even with a comprehensive package of support services.

Several studies have found that those carers who are experiencing psychological problems, but who have kept an open mind about residential care, experience a lessening of their symptoms after the patient is placed.

8.20 What should I consider when choosing a home?

The local Social Services department can provide a list of homes in an area. It is important to note that not all homes can manage patients with dementia. Those designated EMI (elderly mentally infirm) will have greater expertise in this area than non-EMI residential homes. Clearly, the skills and attitudes of the carers and managers are vital and these should be checked by visiting the home, talking to the staff and observing them at work.

Look for evidence of a programme of activities and outings, and access to a garden. A single room might be preferred to a shared one. In any case, the room should be large enough for comfort and to accommodate some furniture. The location of the home will be an important consideration if your relative has strong ties with a specific town or village, and if relatives or friends are likely to be visiting regularly.

Dementia, ethics and the law

9

9.1   What ethical and legal issues affect patients with dementia?

Patients with dementia frequently lack specific abilities, judgement and understanding. There are many situations in which the need to ensure wellbeing, financial security or safety conflict with the rights or wishes of a hitherto autonomous adult. This chapter addresses the various areas of statute law relevant to patients with dementia, such as the Mental Health Act (England and Wales only) and regulations relating to driving (the whole of the UK). It also provides practical advice on assessing capacity for consent, how to act in the patient's 'best interests' and how to ensure that a patient's financial interests are safeguarded.

The answers to the following questions are written from a UK perspective; the general principles apply more broadly.

DRIVING

9.2   Should patients with dementia drive?

There is no simple answer to this question. Some patients will be so impaired that they are obviously unsafe behind the wheel and therefore should not drive. But driving is a learned skill and becomes almost automatic. Patients with quite a marked degree of cognitive impairment seem to be able to drive competently, so long as they stick to familiar routes and nothing untoward occurs during the journey. However, should the driver need to take avoiding action or perform an unfamiliar manoeuvre then lack of skill, slow reflexes or poor judgement might be highlighted. Patients who have lost all awareness of the extent of their difficulties are likely to be particularly unsafe behind the wheel.

Possible problems with driving should be part of any dementia assessment. However, patients are often very sensitive about suggestions that their driving skills might be impaired. The possibility of losing a licence can cause significant distress because it threatens loss of independence and significant inconvenience, particularly in rural areas.

9.3   What is the law concerning patients with dementia driving?

It is the responsibility of the licence holder to notify the DVLA of any psychiatric condition that is relapsing, recurrent or progressive and which may make the driver a source of danger. The DVLA must therefore be informed of a diagnosis of dementia. This notification should occur immediately after diagnosis. If a licence is not revoked, disclosure is necessary on renewal of the licence at the driver's 70th birthday, and at renewal every 3 years thereafter.

A diagnosis of dementia does not inevitably lead to a loss of licence. A licence can be issued (or not revoked) subject to yearly review in cases of early dementia where driving skills are retained and progression of the disease is slow. Medical reports are requested and a formal driving assessment is sometimes required.

According to the DVLA, 'impairment of cognitive functioning is not usually compatible with the driving of [group 2] vehicles', i.e. lorries and buses.

9.4 Who decides whether patients with dementia can drive?

It is the licence holder's responsibility to inform the DVLA (www.dvla.gov.uk). Ultimately, the DVLA's medical adviser decides whether a licence should be revoked. However, a patient with dementia might not be able, or might refuse, to notify the DVLA and carries on driving. In these circumstances, according to the GMC, a doctor has a duty to:

- inform the DVLA immediately if patient cannot understand advice that driving ability might be affected
- make every effort to persuade patient to stop, e.g. inform next of kin
- disclose relevant medical information to the medical adviser at the DVLA.

Before giving medical information to the DVLA, the patient should be notified and then informed in writing to confirm that disclosure has occurred.

If a patient continues to drive after the licence has been revoked, it might be necessary to inform family members and suggest that they perhaps immobilize or remove the car. If there is clear risk of serious danger to other road users, a doctor might have to consider breaching medical confidentiality and notify the Police.

9.5 Are any facilities available to assess a patient's driving ability?

There are a number of disabled drivers' assessment centres throughout England and Wales. They provide a comprehensive assessment of fitness to drive, including physical and visual evaluation, cognitive and perceptual assessment and testing using both static simulators and real cars. There is a list of centres in the back of the document published by the DVLA entitled *At-a-glance guide to the current medical standards of fitness to drive.*

MEDICAL TREATMENT AND CONSENT

9.6 My patient has dementia and is refusing to go into hospital for life-saving medical treatment. What should I do?

First, it is necessary to establish the patient's capacity for consent. Despite having dementia, an individual might have sufficient cognitive function to appraise the situation and reach a reasoned decision. If a patient who has capacity to consent chooses not to accept treatment this decision should be respected, even if, as a doctor, one disagreed with it. It would be unlawful and unethical to attempt to enforce treatment, although it might be appropriate to continue to try to persuade the patient to accept the treatment.

If a patient does not have sufficient capacity to consent a doctor must then act in the 'best interests' of the patient. In this case, it might be reasonable not to take 'no' for an answer and to insist on admission. And ambulance personnel are often very persuasive. Nevertheless, unreasonable force should never be used and, in practice, there are many examples of treatment (such as giving medication by mouth) that cannot be administered without some cooperation from the patient.

However, acting in the 'best interests' of a patient might also involve deciding not to submit the patient to invasive, uncomfortable or unnecessary investigations and treatment. It might be agreed, after consultation with the patient and family members, that active medical treatment would serve no useful purpose.

9.7 Can a next of kin or spouse give consent on behalf of a patient with dementia?

No. It is important to take the views of family members into account but neither the spouse nor next of kin (nor anyone else) has the legal power to give, or withhold, consent for medical treatment on an adult patient's behalf. This applies irrespective of the patient's mental capacity or physical condition.

9.8 How do I assess capacity for consent?

It is the responsibility of any doctor treating a patient to ensure that the patient has the capacity to give valid consent. Patients are assumed to be able to give (or withhold) consent unless proven otherwise. The presence of mental disorder or dementia does not in itself determine whether or not a person lacks capacity. In determining capacity to consent to treatment, a doctor must ensure that a patient:

- can understand and retain the information relevant to the decision in question
- believes the information he has been given
- is able to weigh that information in the balance and arrive at a choice.

Capacity can fluctuate. All efforts should be made to maximize capacity, for example by providing aids to communication and conducting the interview in such a way as to reduce anxiety as much as possible. If the incapacity is temporary because of an episode of delirium, the assessment should be delayed until the medical condition improves.

Each assessment of capacity has to be done with the specific function or decision in mind. Different levels of capacity are required for different activities. A person might have the capacity to consent to a relatively straightforward course of action, e.g. changing dressings, but not have the capacity to consent to a complex and risky surgical procedure.

9.9 What should a patient be able to do to have capacity?

To demonstrate capacity, a patient should:

- understand the nature and purpose of the proposed treatment
- understand its benefits, possible adverse effects and alternatives
- understand the implications of refusing the proposed treatment
- retain the information for long enough to make a decision
- make a choice free from coercion or pressure.

Although the patient might arrive at a decision that could be considered irrational, this does not necessarily mean the patient therefore lacks the capacity to consent.

9.10 What does 'best interests' mean?

Some types of treatment remain lawful even in the absence of the patient's consent. The procedures have to be deemed 'necessary'. In this context, 'necessity' can be defined as:

- there must be a necessity to act despite consent not being available
- the action taken must be what a reasonable person would take in the same circumstances. In the case of medical treatment, it is expected that a doctor would act in a way that would be considered accepted (but not necessarily 'standard') practice by a responsible and competent body of relevant professional opinion.

9.11 How do I determine what is in the best interests of my patient?

When determining what action to take, consideration must be given to:

- any known past and present wishes of the individual
- maximizing as far as possible the individual's participation in the process
- the views of others (e.g. family) as to the person's wishes and feelings
- the need to take the course of action that is least restrictive of the person's freedom.

'Best interests' does not apply only to emergency situations and can be extended to forms of health care, including routine, but essential, nursing that is intended to ensure improvement or prevent deterioration of health.

Not only are doctors able to provide treatment in these circumstances, they have a duty of care to do so. However, it would not be lawful to proceed with treatment that a patient, when of sound mind, had formally stated objections to, for example in an advanced directive.

THE MENTAL HEALTH ACT

9.12 What about the Mental Health Act?

Patients with dementia do not always understand, if they have a life-threatening medical condition, the necessity of admission and treatment. However, it is not legal to use the Mental Health Act to compel them to go to hospital for treatment of that medical condition.

The Mental Health Act (MHA) of England and Wales (1983) provides a legal mechanism for admitting patients without their consent for assessment and/or treatment of *a mental disorder* (not a physical condition). Certain criteria need to be met regarding the nature or degree of the mental disorder and the reasons for the admission. The admission must be in the interests of the patient's health or safety and/or for the protection of others. The act provides safeguards to the patient's civil liberties in the form of conditions and procedures for compulsory admission, mechanisms for appeal against detention in hospital, and implementation of independent reviews of treatment.

9.13 How is the Mental Health Act used with patients with dementia?

The terms 'mental illness' or 'mental disorder' in the context of the MHA are open to some interpretation but the definitions include dementia, despite the fact that dementia is an organic brain disease.

A patient with dementia might require urgent psychiatric admission in a number of circumstances. In most cases there will be concern about the individual's safety at home, which could result in deterioration of the patient's health (both mental and physical) or a safety risk. The patient might be incapable of preparing meals yet refusing support at home and, as a result, becoming malnourished and dehydrated. Or the patient might be repeatedly wandering out of home at night in all weathers, and therefore at risk of hypothermia, injury from falls or assault. There could be a risk to others as a result of the onset or worsening of aggressive behaviour.

9.14 How is an admission under the Mental Health Act organized?

Attempts would first be made to implement suitable home care or other support and monitoring services. If this is deemed inadequate or if the patient refuses, an admission for assessment and to provide a place of safety would be considered. Every attempt should first be made to persuade the patient to come in voluntarily. If this is not successful then an MHA assessment is arranged between the GP, an 'approved' social worker and a senior psychiatrist, all of whom must agree that the grounds for admission have been met.

A patient whose diagnosis is not known, is unclear or in whom there has been an acute change in symptoms or behaviour can be admitted for assessment under Section 2 of the MHA. This lasts up to 28 days. If admission under the MHA is required beyond this time, a treatment order – Section 3 – must be implemented. This lasts 6 months and can be renewed thereafter. Although dementia is not a 'treatable' condition in the conventional medical sense of the word, 'treatment' in the context of the MHA includes nursing care as well as medication used, for example, to control agitated or aggressive behaviour.

9.15 Do all patients with dementia requiring psychiatric admission need the Mental Health Act?

At the time of writing it is not the convention to implement the MHA for every patient with dementia requiring psychiatric admission. Patients can be admitted and receive necessary treatment 'voluntarily' despite not having full capacity to consent, as long as they seem to have some understanding of their circumstances and demonstrate passive consent. 'Passive consent' means that the patient accepts the admission and any treatment without verbal dissent or demonstrating dissent in other ways (e.g. struggling, attempting to leave).

9.16 What is 'guardianship'?

Patients might not need admission to hospital but still require measures to be taken to ensure their safety and welfare. The MHA allows for this under the guardianship order. A patient must be suffering from mental illness or severe mental impairment of a nature or degree as to necessitate reception into guardianship. This initially lasts 6 months but can be renewed. The guardian, which is usually the local social services authority, but can be a relative, has the power to:

- require the patient to live in a specified place
- require the patient to attend for treatment, reassessment and so on at specified places and at specified times; but treatment cannot be enforced

■ require access to the patient to be given to doctors, social workers and other clinical staff (e.g. community nurses involved in the patient's care).

For a guardianship order to be effective, the patient has to cooperate. For example, the order does not give authority for patients to be physically removed from their home against their will. For this reason, this part of the MHA is infrequently used.

9.17   What is Section 47 of the National Assistance Act?

Section 47 of the National Assistance Act provides the power to remove elderly people from their homes and place them in hospital or institutional care if they are demonstrating severe neglect, living in squalid and insanitary conditions and refusing the necessary support. They must be aged and infirm, being physically incapacitated or suffering from chronic physical disease, but not necessarily mentally disordered. An application is usually requested by the GP or psychiatrist and made by a public health physician, through the magistrates court. However, it is rarely used nowadays out of concern that the process affords insufficient protection to the patient's civil liberties.

9.18   What are the potential implications of the new Mental Health Act?

The proposals for the new Mental Health Act, which, at the time of writing, is currently the subject of a Parliamentary Bill have certain implications for those involved in the care of patients with dementia.

It has been accepted that those patients who are 'passively consenting' to their admission need not be subject to detention under the MHA even though, by virtue of their dementia, they are unable to give informed consent. By remaining 'voluntary' patients they do not have the safeguards that ensure that patients detained under the MHA are not admitted or treated inappropriately. These safeguards include the right to appeal to a mental health tribunal and monitoring of treatment by the Mental Health Act Commission via 'second opinion approved doctors'.

The draft new Mental Health Act indicates that although such patients can remain in hospital without formal detention, their care should still undergo independent review. It proposes that care plans for all patients will be drawn up in respect of the patients' medical, nursing and social management and submitted to an independent Mental Health Act Commission for scrutiny and ratification. Such care plans are used routinely in hospitals but not in residential or nursing homes. It has been proposed that the system so described should apply to patients in these settings as well as in hospital.

Independent reviews of care of patients in care homes are welcomed. What is not yet clear is whether there will be sufficient clinicians available to adopt the system.

FINANCES

9.19 How can a patient's financial affairs be safeguarded?

Patients with moderate or severe dementia are likely to have problems managing their financial affairs. In many cases this is dealt with informally, perhaps by a neighbour collecting the pension and a son or daughter paying the bills. Patients often carry on signing cheques, under supervision, even when not fully aware of what they are doing. Clearly, this arrangement will not be satisfactory in the longer term. There are two main ways in which a patient's financial affairs can be put on a more formal footing: appointeeship and enduring power of attorney.

9.20 What is 'appointeeship'?

Appointeeship allows for another person to claim, receive and spend state benefits on the behalf of someone who is deemed to be incapable of managing his or her financial affairs. An appointee, who might be a social worker or family member, is limited to managing state benefit income. Appointeeship is therefore insufficient where financial affairs are complex or if a house needs to be sold to fund residential care.

9.21 What is a 'power of attorney' and 'enduring power of attorney'?

Any competent individual (donor) can appoint someone else (attorney) to act on his or her behalf in relation to his or her financial affairs (power of attorney). However, this becomes invalid if that individual subsequently becomes mentally incapable of managing and administering his or her financial affairs. An enduring power of attorney (EPA) allows for this power to be continued even after someone becomes mentally incapable. When this occurs, the EPA must be registered with the Court of Protection, whose function it is (via the Public Trust Office) to oversee the management of the mentally incapable donor's financial affairs. The Court of Protection can, for example, displace an unsatisfactory attorney.

9.22 What level of understanding is needed to make a valid enduring power of attorney?

Four pieces of information are necessary for a donor to understand when making an enduring power of attorney (EPA):

- that the appointed attorney will have complete authority over the donor's affairs, unless the EPA has been specifically restricted
- that the attorney will be able to do anything with the donor's property that the donor would have done (unless, again, specific restrictions have been imposed)
- that the authority will continue if the donor should be, or should become, mentally incapable
- that should the donor become mentally incapable, that power of the EPA can be revoked only through the Court of Protection.

9.23 How do I assess capacity to manage financial affairs?

Less mental capacity is needed to cope with limited and simple financial affairs – collecting pension, paying rent and so on – than is needed to manage more complex financial matters like investments and property management. The patient's financial needs and responsibilities must be taken into account, as must any likely changes in the patient's circumstances in the future. Other factors to be considered include the extent of available support, the likelihood of the patient making inappropriate financial decisions and how vulnerable the patient is to exploitation.

OTHER LEGAL ISSUES

9.24 What is 'testamentary capacity'?

Testamentary capacity is the degree of understanding required in law to make a valid will. Where there is doubt as to testamentary capacity, solicitors often seek a doctor's advice. When assessing testamentary capacity, as in other forms of capacity, it is the ability to make the decision that is being assessed and not how wise, sensible or morally right that decision is.

9.25 What is required to make a valid will?

To make a valid will, a patient must:

- understand what a will is and the consequences and implications of making a will
- have a realistic understanding of the extent of the assets
- know to whom the assets are bequeathed and know who else might have a just claim on them
- not be suffering from a mental abnormality that affects judgement relating to the disposal of the estate.

Legally revoking an existing will requires a similar level of capacity.

9.26 Can people with dementia marry?

Yes. All a person needs to demonstrate is a broad understanding of the duties and responsibilities of marriage. However, either party might subsequently petition for the marriage to be annulled. It has to be shown that mental disorder at the time of the marriage made a spouse incapable of living in a married state, and carrying out the duties and obligations of marriage.

9.27 What crimes do people with dementia commit?

Causes of criminal behaviour in patients with dementia include sexual disinhibition, (exposure, indecent assault); lack of judgement (shoplifting, driving offences); agitation and aggression (breach of peace, assault). A small minority of cases reach court.

 PATIENT QUESTIONS

9.28 Are people with dementia more likely to crash their car?

On an individual basis, people with significant cognitive impairment are more likely to be at risk of being involved in a car crash. They are also more likely to suffer a fatal injury because they are more likely to be elderly and frail. On the other hand, older patients with dementia drive fewer miles and usually restrict themselves to familiar routes. So it is likely that overall the risk is only slightly increased.

9.29 The nurse in charge of the local nursing home tells me she often puts sedative medication in the residents' tea. Is this ethical?

The routine use of medication given in this (covert) way is unethical. The use of sedative medication is occasionally necessary to prevent behavioural disturbance escalating to the point where patients or staff are at risk. In these situations, a nurse acting in the best interests of an incompetent patient might decide that putting a sedative drug in tea or in a sandwich is the only possible way of ensuring that the patient receives necessary medication. It is important that the nurse documents these actions and it is also good practice to inform the patient's next of kin or close relative.

The excessive use of sedative medication in residential care settings is a cause for concern. Such prescriptions should be closely monitored by the patient's GP.

Alzheimer's disease

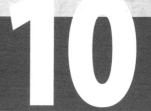

10

10.1 What is Alzheimer's disease?

Alzheimer's disease is the most common cause of dementia in the Western world; it accounts for 50–60 % of all cases of dementia. Until relatively recently it was assumed to be an almost inevitable aspect of ageing and, consequently, attracted little interest. However, the last decade has seen significant advances in our understanding of the pathological, neurochemical and genetic processes involved in this condition. This work has contributed to the development of medication specifically licensed for use in patients with Alzheimer's disease. The scientific interest shown in this condition has been paralleled by the gradual acceptance by the general public that Alzheimer's disease is a medical condition. Stigma is lessening, thanks largely to the efforts of Alzheimer's associations and charities such as the Alzheimer's Society (in the UK) and Alzheimer's Disease International (ADI).

10.2 Why is it called Alzheimer's disease?

Initially, the term 'Alzheimer's disease' was used to describe severe presenile degenerative dementia. In 1907, Alois Alzheimer reported the case of a 51-year-old woman with progressive memory impairment, psychotic symptoms and behavioural disturbance. At postmortem her brain showed plaques and tangles, and signs of cerebrovascular disease. This was significant because it showed that pathology already associated with senile dementia could and did occur in younger patients, causing very similar symptoms. Senile dementia could no longer be ascribed simply to the effects of ageing. It became clear that presenile and senile forms of the disease could not reliably be differentiated on clinical or pathological grounds. So the term 'Alzheimer's disease' became used irrespective of the age of the patient.

PREVALENCE

10.3 How common is Alzheimer's disease?

Alzheimer's disease is the most common cause of dementia in Europe and North America, accounting for about 60% of cases. Around 500 000 people in England and Wales have Alzheimer's disease. The number of affected individuals increases with age, with slightly more women than men developing the condition.

10.4 What is the prevalence according to age?

A rough guide, with figures representing cases per 100 population, is:

- under 70 years of age: 0.5
- 70–80 years of age: 3
- Over 80%: 11.

Put another way: of all cases of Alzheimer's disease:

- 5% will be under 70 years
- 30% will be aged between 70 and 80 years
- 65% will be over 80 years.

SYMPTOMS OF ALZHEIMER'S DISEASE

10.5 What is the typical presentation of Alzheimer's disease?

Patients typically present with memory loss for recent events and for recently acquired information (*Box 10.1*). Longer-term or autobiographical memory is usually preserved at this stage. It is frequently a spouse, relative or carer who seeks medical advice, and not the person concerned, who might be relatively unaware of the difficulties. It is likely that the informant has noticed steadily worsening memory over several months or years. Initially, this might not cause problems but, as it gets worse, the sufferer will mislay items, miss appointments, forget to take medication, and so on, which then prompts the carer to seek help. Such problems can be compounded by a degree of disorientation in time or place.

A patient in the early stages of the condition can become less articulate and fluent, and have difficulty with word finding. It might also be apparent that the patient's ability to learn new skills is affected. The patient might remain self-caring but the skill required to engage in more complex motor activities, particularly those that are not part of a daily routine, will be impaired.

A patient often loses the motivation, initiative or confidence to perform a daily activity that was previously familiar to them. The spouse might complain of having to repeatedly remind the sufferer to do things, or being required to take on more of the household tasks. In such cases, the onset of Alzheimer's disease can be mistaken for depression.

LOSS OF FUNCTIONAL ABILITY

10.6 What symptoms develop as Alzheimer's disease progresses?

Memory and language function deteriorate further. Conversation becomes stilted and superficial and the patient might become increasingly repetitive.

> **Box 10.1 Summary of the main clinical features of Alzheimer's disease**
> - Memory loss, initially for recent events
> - Language impairment
> - Decline in complex motor skills
> - Disorientation
> - Loss of recognition skills

Understanding of written material declines, as do reading and writing skills and the ability to perform calculations or mental arithmetic. Difficulties in managing finances can result. Sufferers are likely to show disorientation in both time and place, often being described as 'living in the past'. Recognition of objects and of familiar faces is often lost; the latter causes particular distress to loved ones.

Visuospatial and motor ability decline, as do ability to sequence and plan tasks. This leads to problems, even with fairly routine and simple daily skills including self-care. Loss of hygiene might be noticeable to all but the individual concerned. Trying to cook can result in the risk of fire and explosion; flooding is a risk when taps are turned on and then forgotten; burning cigarettes can be mislaid. The patient might get lost returning from a walk to the local shops.

10.7 What is a typical presentation for Alzheimer's disease?

CASE STUDY

Vera Creake is an 83-year-old widow. She is fit for her age with no significant medical conditions. Her conversation has become repetitive and she has missed two doctor's appointments recently. She acknowledges that her memory is 'not what it was' but denies that it causes problems and puts it down to her age. Although Mrs Creake still copes fairly well on her own, her daughter has noticed that her home has become rather less tidy and she has often found food in her fridge that has exceeded the sell-by-date. Mrs Creake has lost some weight and her daughter suspects that she sometimes forgets to eat.

10.8 How quickly does the condition progress?

The time from onset to diagnosis is usually 1 to 2 years. Although the condition is progressive, deterioration varies widely. Patients might show relatively mild decline for several years before more dramatic deterioration takes place. As a rule, a decline of 4 points per year on the MMSE score is expected. Around 10% of cases experience plateaux where there is no significant deterioration for several years.

10.9 What symptoms occur in the later stages of the disease?

Language function deteriorates to the point that all coherent speech is lost. Eventually, this can lead to a state of virtual mutism. There is loss of recognition of surroundings, people and commonplace objects. Functional ability declines to the stage where the patient requires assistance with all aspects of self-care, including feeding and toileting. It is in the later stages that physical signs and symptoms supervene.

10.10 What physical symptoms occur in patients with Alzheimer's disease?

Epileptic seizures are fairly common (in at least 10% of patients), especially in the later stages of Alzheimer's disease. Gait apraxia results in unsteadiness and greater risk of falls. This can be associated with extrapyramidal (parkinsonian) signs, particularly muscle rigidity and bradykinesia (slowness of movement).

Appetite and the ability to master the mechanics of eating are impaired. The result is loss of weight and problems associated with malnutrition and dehydration, increased susceptibility to infection, osteoporosis and vitamin deficiency.

As the disease reaches its later stages, the patient becomes increasingly immobile and, ultimately, bed- or chairbound. Other physical symptoms are a consequence of immobility and include contractures, pressure sores, and orthostatic pneumonia.

10.11 Should seizures be treated in patients with advanced Alzheimer's disease?

A single seizure or episodes that are not clearly epileptiform are best not treated. Instead, the situation should be monitored. If seizures become frequent, treatment with anticonvulsants is indicated. Carbamazepine is a suitable choice, although valproate is an alternative.

10.12 What psychotic symptoms occur?

It is during the middle phase that the neuropsychiatric and behavioural manifestations of Alzheimer's disease typically occur. Visual hallucinations occur in one-fifth of patients and are particularly common if there is coexisting visual impairment due to cataract or macular degeneration. Patients often report seeing people in the house who should not be there. They are vivid and lifelike and can cause distress.

Delusions or abnormal beliefs occur, triggered by a degree of suspicion combined with the memory loss or functional impairment itself. For example, patients might accuse a relative or carer of stealing valuables when in fact they have been put in an unusual, and quickly forgotten, hiding place. Or patients might believe that someone has broken in and interfered with belongings and furniture when, of course, the disarray is a direct consequence of their problems coping with daily household chores. Sometimes they phone the Police. Such symptoms, when there is also some loss of emotional control, often result in distress and agitation.

10.13 What is the implication of onset of psychotic symptoms?

Persistent psychotic symptoms often cause distress, agitation or other behavioural problems. Delusions can lead directly to confrontational behaviour, such as falsely accusing neighbours. Patients with psychotic symptoms as well as Alzheimer's disease are more likely to be admitted to hospital or residential care. It might also indicate a more rapid deterioration of the dementing illness.

The sudden onset of psychotic symptoms can indicate the development of delirium (*see Qs 1.21–1.23*). The possibility of infection or other acute illness, or adverse effects of recently prescribed medication, should be considered.

10.14 What causes agitation?

Psychotic symptoms frequently cause agitation. Another cause of agitation is severe disorientation leading to loss of recognition that the patient is in his or her own home. This results in repeated requests to 'go home', packing cases and trying to leave the house at inappropriate times of day (and often inappropriately dressed). Attempts to rationalize or restrain usually make the agitation worse and can result in verbal or physical aggression. Wandering is less purposeful but equally difficult for a carer to manage, particularly as it is often associated with disturbance of the sleep/wake cycle and disorientation in time, resulting in severe nocturnal restlessness.

10.15 What are the implications of agitation and other behavioural disturbances?

Behavioural disturbance correlates with the severity of dementia and is more likely to cause carer burden than the cognitive impairment itself. Patients who display behavioural disturbance are more likely to be placed in residential care or require hospital admission. Agitation and wandering increase the risk of falls and subsequent injury.

10.16 Can physical aggression be predicted?

Physical aggression occurs in about 20% of patients with Alzheimer's disease. A history of aggressive behaviour that predates the onset of dementia and a poor relationship with spouse or carer both increase the risks of aggression. Physical illness or psychological problems, such as depression or anxiety, can trigger a sudden increase of physical aggression. The onset of psychotic symptoms, such as visual hallucinations or persecutory delusions, must also be considered as a contributory factor. Environmental factors might include changes in routine, care staff, or location.

10.17 What are the effects of loss of insight?

In this context, insight is the conscious awareness of one's own illness, including its symptoms and its implications for oneself and others. Insight is reduced in the relatively early stages of Alzheimer's disease. Patients, therefore, might have little idea that they are not coping as well as they used to, or that their behaviour is becoming potentially risky or antisocial. In these circumstances it can be difficult to persuade a sufferer to accept home help, take medication or agree to move into residential care.

However, reduction of insight does not necessarily mean that patients have no idea that they are having difficulties. A realization that 'something is wrong but I don't know what' often results in frustration and irritability, and is likely to increase the risk of agitation and aggression.

10.18 Which symptoms point to a diagnosis of Alzheimer's disease?

In many ways, the diagnosis of Alzheimer's disease is one of exclusion. Diagnostic criteria require the absence of other brain or systemic disorders that might be contributing to the dementia, such as severe cerebrovascular disease.

DIAGNOSING ALZHEIMER'S DISEASE

10.19 What are the diagnostic criteria for Alzheimer's disease?

The McKhann (National Institute for Neurological and Communicative Disorders and Stroke (and the) Alzheimer's Disease and Related Disorders Association; NINCDS–ADRDA) diagnostic criteria are shown in *Box 10.2*.

10.20 Can any physical investigations or tests confirm the diagnosis?

Currently, no diagnostic investigations can provide confirmation of the disease; all investigations are performed to exclude secondary causes of dementia.

However, CT or MRI imaging techniques, which allow for the measurement of the medial temporal lobe and hippocampus, now exist; focal atrophy of this brain region is specifically associated with Alzheimer's disease. A computer technique has also been developed that allows for the precise alignment of sequential MRI scans over a period of time. The loss of brain tissue from one scan to another can then be visualized and measured. Potentially, therefore, progressive but subtle cortical atrophy can be identified at a very early stage, before major cognitive impairment becomes evident. These two techniques are still in the research stage.

Imaging can show relatively focal atrophy of the temporal lobes including the hippocampus (*Fig. 10.1*) or more diffuse atrophy (*Fig. 10.2*). Diffuse atrophy might be more apparent on coronal sections (*Fig. 10.3*).

10.21 What parts of the brain are affected by Alzheimer's disease?

Cholinergic neurons are specifically affected in the basal nuclei, including the locus coeruleus, hippocampus and the entorrhinal cortex. Nerve cell

---

Box 10.2 The McKhann (NINCDS-ADRDA) criteria for diagnosing Alzheimer's disease (McKhann et al 1984)

For the diagnosis of *probable* Alzheimer's disease:

- Dementia established by clinical examination and rating scales or neuropsychological tests
- Deficits in two or more areas of cognition
- Progressive worsening of memory and other cognitive functions
- No disturbance of consciousness
- Onset between 40 and 90 years
- Absence of systemic disorders of other brain diseases to account for the symptoms of dementia

The diagnosis is *supported by*:

- Progressive deterioration of specific cognitive functions such as language, motor skills and perception
- Impaired activities of daily living and altered patterns of behaviour
- Family history of similar disorder, particularly if confirmed neuropathologically
- Evidence of cortical atrophy on CT with progression on serial scanning
- Non-specific EEG changes only
- Normal CSF

Other features consistent with diagnosis are:

- Plateaux in the clinical course
- Associated neuropsychiatric symptoms including depression, hallucinations, delusions, incontinence, insomnia
- Seizures in advanced disease
- CT brain scan might be normal for age

Features making diagnosis *unlikely are*:

- Sudden onset
- Focal neurological signs eg hemiparesis, visual field defects, incoordination in early stage
- Seizures or gait disturbance at onset or early in course of disease

A diagnosis of *definite* Alzheimer's disease:

- A definite diagnosis can only be made on identification of histopathological evidence obtained from biopsy or autopsy. However using these criteria enables a diagnostic accuracy of around 80%

---

loss causing cerebral atrophy is most pronounced in the (medial) temporal and frontal lobes. As the disease progresses, all areas of the cortex become involved, although the occipital cortex is relatively spared

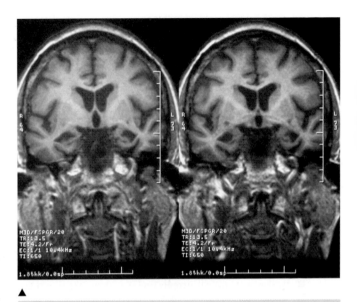

▲

Fig. 10.1 Severe temporal lobe atrophy including the hippocampi seen on an MRI scan in a patient with clinical Alzheimer's disease.

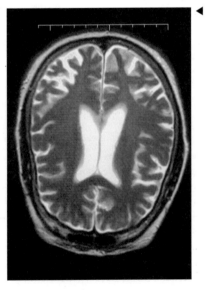

◄ **Fig. 10.2** Diffuse cerebral atrophy shown on an MRI scan in a patient with clinical Alzheimer's disease.

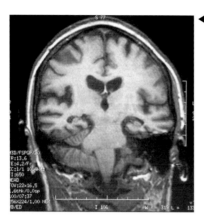

Fig. 10.3 The atrophy is more apparent on coronal sections from the same scan.

AETIOLOGY OF ALZHEIMER'S DISEASE

10.22 What causes Alzheimer's disease?

The best current theory is that Alzheimer's disease is associated with deposition of a protein called beta-amyloid in and around nerve cells of the brain. The lateral parts of the brain – the temporal lobes – are usually affected first. Beta-amyloid is formed from a normal body protein called amyloid precursor protein (APP), whose function is as yet unknown. In certain individuals, as a result of abnormal processing of the APP, excess quantities of beta-amyloid are produced. Beta-amyloid aggregates, forming plaques within the neuronal tissue of the cerebral cortex. Amyloid deposits are also formed in the cerebral arterioles.

Other cerebral pathology found in the brains of Alzheimer's patients are intracellular neurofibrillary tangles. These are formed from abnormally phosphorylated protein (tau protein), which disrupts cellular architecture and its consequent functioning. Markers of the inflammatory process – microglia and astrocytes – are also found and it is believed that they are closely associated with the formation of the plaques and tangles.

Further support for the role of the inflammatory process is found in the epidemiological evidence suggesting that there are links between the long-term use of non-steroidal anti-inflammatory drugs and a reduced risk of developing Alzheimer's disease.

10.23 Does aluminium cause Alzheimer's disease?

It is possible that exposure to excess quantities of aluminium is one factor that contributes to the development of Alzheimer's disease. However, it is very unlikely that the use of aluminium saucepans or deodorants represents a risk.

Various epidemiological studies have found an association between prevalence of Alzheimer's disease and the level of aluminium in drinking water. Animal studies have shown that intracerebral injections of aluminium salts can trigger the formation of Alzheimer-type pathology and microscopic foci of aluminium have been found in amyloid plaques in the brains of human sufferers. So-called 'dialysis dementia' or encephalopathy can occur after renal haemodialysis. The condition is associated with higher than normal aluminium deposits in the brain and is believed to be a result of the aluminium content of the water used in the procedure.

10.24 What environmental factors cause Alzheimer's disease?

Apart from aluminium, other possible environmental factors implicated in the development of Alzheimer's disease include head injury and infection.

Severe head injury resulting in loss of consciousness is thought to increase the relative risk of developing Alzheimer's disease two-fold. Such trauma is known to trigger an acute intracerebral inflammatory reaction with the formation of astrocytes and microglia. These, in turn, increase amyloid plaque formation.

Herpes simplex virus type 1 infection has been found to be a risk factor but only in individuals with the apolipoprotein E (apo E) e4 allele.

10.25 Do smoking and drinking affect the risk of Alzheimer's disease?

There is no clear evidence for an association between smoking and Alzheimer's disease. Theoretically, smoking might reduce the risk of developing, or even ameliorate, the symptoms of Alzheimer's disease via its effect on nicotinic receptors in the cortex. However, any benefits are likely to be outweighed by the increased cardiovascular and cerebrovascular risks incurred.

There appears to be no association between alcohol consumption and Alzheimer's disease. However, the putative antioxidant properties of red wine have already led to claims of benefit on many aspects of ageing including the development of dementia

GENETICS OF ALZHEIMER'S DISEASE

10.26 Is Alzheimer's disease associated with genetic defects?

Gene mutations at several sites have been identified as potentially causing, or increasing, an individual's risk of developing the disease. These include the gene for amyloid precursor protein (APP) on chromosome 21. The connection with Down syndrome due to trisomy 21 is interesting in this respect: patients with Down syndrome surviving into their 50s are greatly at risk of developing Alzheimer's disease. At chromosome 21, abnormal coding for amyloid precursor protein results in excessive deposition of beta-amyloid, resulting in plaque formation.

The so-called presenilin genes (presenilin 1 and 2) are associated with gene mutations on chromosomes 14 and 1, respectively. When both are present, they are thought to account for a significant number of cases (about 50%) of early-onset Alzheimer's disease but only a tiny proportion of cases overall. It is likely that other gene mutations will be identified.

10.27 What are the characteristic features of genetically inherited Alzheimer's disease?

- Onset between the ages of 40 and 60 years.
- Autosomal dominant inheritance.
- Seizures.
- Myoclonus.

10.28 What is apo E?

Apolipoprotein E (apo E) is involved in intracellular transport and metabolism of cholesterol and other lipids. As such, it is believed to play a part in amyloid deposition. The gene that encodes for apo E is on chromosome 19 and has three alleles: apo E2, apo E3 and apo E4. An individual's apo E genotype will comprise a pair of alleles, each of which could be apo E2, 3 or 4.

Apo E4 appears to increase vulnerability rather than being a causative agent itself. The risk of developing Alzheimer's disease is increased significantly (up to 30 times) if a patient is homozygous for apo E4, (i.e. if both of the pair are apo E4) and the age at onset decreases if an individual has one or more apo E4 alleles.

Individuals with the E2 allele, either homozygously or in combination with the E3 allele, appear to have a reduced risk of developing the disease.

10.29 Is genetic screening helpful?

Yes, in autosomal dominant variants. Early-onset Alzheimer's disease is more closely associated with identified single gene abnormalities (presenilin, amyloid precursor protein). It is likely to be inherited in an autosomal dominant manner, i.e. the child of a sufferer has a 50% chance of developing the disease. Genetic testing can therefore not only help diagnosis but also permit unaffected family members to seek genetic counselling. Later-onset Alzheimer's disease is rarely associated with single gene defects. There is no indication currently to perform genetic testing in these cases.

Apo E status does appear to be a definite marker of biological risk in late onset Alzheimer's disease. However, it only indicates risk. Patients can be homozygous for apo E4 and not develop the disease, and many patients with the disease do not have the genes that suggest a risk. Therefore, although this line of research raises the possibility of early diagnosis and prediction, routine testing for apo E is not yet indicated for later-onset Alzheimer's disease.

10.30 Who should be tested for genetic risk factors?

Diagnostic testing might be appropriate in cases of suspected familial early-onset Alzheimer's disease. Predictive testing of at risk family members should also be considered. DNA banking might be an option where there is real concern over risk but a family member is reluctant to proceed with testing, or where an affected family member is not available to test first. In any case, it is recommended that advice is sought from a regional genetics department or the Alzheimer's Disease Genetics Consortium.

ALZHEIMER'S DISEASE AND DEATH

10.31 What is the life expectancy?

On average, time from diagnosis to death is about 8 years. Life expectancy is, therefore shortened in patients with Alzheimer's disease. But this varies greatly (from 2 to 20 years from onset of the disease) and depends on the age at onset and the rate of progression. Exact predictions are not possible, not least because the onset of the disease itself can rarely be accurately dated. Women appear to have a better life expectancy than men.

Patients who have difficulty with their food or fluid intake are clearly more at risk from the effects of malnutrition and dehydration. Agitation and risk-taking behaviour will increase the risk of falls, head injury and fractures, which will all influence prognosis. Persistent psychotic symptoms also indicate poor prognosis.

10.32 What do patients with Alzheimer's disease die from?

The most common cause of death in patients with Alzheimer's disease is bronchopneumonia, followed by cardiovascular disease and pulmonary embolism. However, this is rarely confirmed by postmortem examination.

Patients with Alzheimer's disease usually die in institutional care. Most are virtually immobile and many have suffered severe weight loss.

PATIENT QUESTIONS

10.33 Do you recommend taking non-steroidal anti-inflammatory drugs, hormone replacement therapy or vitamin E supplements to help prevent Alzheimer's disease?

Although the research findings look promising there is insufficient evidence to recommend taking drugs, hormones or vitamin supplements as a preventive measure.

10.34 My mother had Alzheimer's disease. Does this increase the chance of me developing the disease?

Parents can be blamed for most things and the short answer is 'Yes'. The risk to first-degree relatives (i.e. children, brothers or sisters) increases with age (as it does for everybody), rising to nearly 50% at 90 years, compared with a risk of 20–30% if there is no family history. However, at that age most people will have already succumbed to something else. It might be reassuring to note that Alzheimer's disease occurring at such an advanced age progresses quite slowly and causes fewer problems compared with the disease in younger people.

Some much rarer forms of Alzheimer's disease, notably the early-onset types, are more obviously inherited and are described as 'autosomal dominant'. In such families, the risk of developing the disease – irrespective of age – will be up to 50%, depending on age of onset and the type of genetic mutation.

Vascular dementia

11.1 What is vascular dementia?

Vascular dementia is one of the most common forms of dementia, although it is little understood and little researched. As the average age and life expectancy of the population increases, vascular dementia is becoming more common. In many patients who develop it the diagnosis is obvious – the patient is known to have vascular disease and vascular risk factors and then, over a period of years, has several clinical strokes resulting in increasing physical and cognitive handicap. This clinical syndrome is called multi-infarct dementia. There are other forms of vascular dementia in which the diagnosis is less obvious because the clinical course mimics a degenerative dementia. It is important to diagnose vascular dementia early because treatment of vascular risk factors may improve the outlook for the patient.

Many patients have a pure vascular dementia but both vascular disease and Alzheimer's disease become so common in patients over the age of 70, that it is hardly surprising that many patients who develop dementia after this age have clinical and pathological features of both Alzheimer's and vascular dementia. In studies, patients with this 'mixed' form of dementia make up about one-fifth of all patients with dementia.

Vascular dementia is the general name for dementia that is due primarily to disease of the blood vessels supplying the brain. Several forms are recognized. One major distinction, which is important in the investigation and treatment of patients, is whether the disease is primarily one of large arteries (causing multiple infarcts) or smaller perforating arteries and arterioles, causing small vessels disease. The different forms of vascular dementia are:

- Multi-infarct dementia: dementia secondary to two or more strokes. The name should be used only in patients who have had clinical strokes. Generally, as well as affecting memory and other cognitive functions, the strokes produce physical problems such as limb weakness, speech problems and visual field losses.
- Small vessel disease: produces a more gradual syndrome in which the patient slows down mentally and often develops gait and other physical problems. It might or might not be accompanied by clinical strokes or transient ischaemic attacks (TIAs). Patients with small vessel disease often have a recognizable picture in which memory is preserved but accessing it is very slow. Patients who are asked questions reply after a long pause, but do give the correct answer.
- CADASIL (cerebral autosomal dominant arteriopathy with subcortical ischaemic leukoencephalopathy): an inherited form of vascular dementia accompanied by other problems such as migraine (*see* Q 11.13).

■ Cerebral vasculitis: an inflammation of the blood vessels to the brain that produces a rapidly progressive dementia (see Chapter 4).

■ Chronic subdural haematoma: one of the treatable dementias (see Chapter 4).

11.2 What is a typical story for a patient with vascular dementia?

CASE STUDY

George Houghton developed hypertension at the age of 50 years and maturity-onset diabetes at 55. He was overweight and a smoker. At the age of 57 years he awoke one morning with a right hemiparesis and an expressive aphasia. He was admitted to the local hospital and a diagnosis of left middle cerebral artery infarct was made. He made some recovery but was left with a mild weakness and some word-finding difficulties. A year later he began to have occasional episodes of transient visual loss in the left eye, this was diagnosed as amaurosis fugax. He then suffered a mild left-sided stroke that affected his face and hand and his speech became worse. He made a good physical recovery but his wife complained that his memory was poorer. A year later he had a sudden onset of right hemianopia – loss of vision to the right side; following this his memory was much worse. He had some difficulty in understanding speech and, although the function in his right hand was reasonable, he could no longer write fluently.

11.3 What is a typical story for a patient with small vessel disease?

CASE STUDY

Henry Rudham developed hypertension at the age of 40 and was monitored by his GP. He was a smoker. At the age of 58 he began to complain that his memory was poorer and his walking less steady. His wife and colleagues complained that he had lost his drive and that he was forgetful and apathetic. A course of antidepressants made no substantial change. The following year, his walking had declined and he bought a stick. His wife noted that he had difficulty initiating movement but that once he started he was not too bad. For example, it would take him a little while to stand up and start walking but once he 'got into his stride' he was nearly as quick as before. He was much slower mentally, although it was a bit of a family joke that he always got there in the end. At times, he could do complex tasks correctly but slowly. He had been able to do the monthly household accounts in a couple of hours; it now took him a whole day and there were some errors.

11.4 Can you develop dementia after a single stroke?

The answer to this question depends on your definition of dementia (*see Q 1.1*). Some definitions exclude single focal events and stress that the cognitive problems must be progressive; such definitions would exclude cognitive problems from a single stroke. However, it is certainly possible for patients to have severe cognitive difficulties following a single stroke. These strokes are usually of the posterior circulation and tend to include the dominant hippocampus and adjacent cortex or the midbrain, thalami and mammillary bodies. A left thalamic infarct is shown in *Fig. 11.1*. It is very

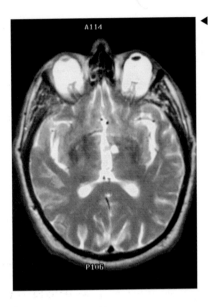

Fig. 11.1 MRI scan showing a left thalamic infarct in a patient with a sudden onset of amnesia.

unusual for a patient to have cognitive problems alone and there are nearly always other features, such as a field defect, speech or motor problem. Many of these patients will make a good recovery in time, although they remain more vulnerable to cognitive problems following further strokes.

11.5 How common is vascular dementia?

It is difficult to obtain good figures for the prevalence of vascular dementia. It depends on how vascular dementia is defined. Post-mortem series suggest that it is the second most common form of dementia after Alzheimer's disease. An estimate would be that about 1–2% of individuals over 70 suffer from a vascular dementia and about the same number again have a mixture of vascular dementia and Alzheimer's disease. This makes it a very common disease.

11.6 Who develops vascular dementia?

Vascular dementia becomes more common with age and with vascular risk factors (*see* Q 11.15). It is more common in men than women and in certain ethnic groups, including individuals of Japanese and Caribbean extraction.

11.7 What parts of the brain are affected by vascular dementia?

All parts of the brain have a blood supply and all can be affected by a stroke. In large vessel disease, strokes affecting the posterior circulation result in memory problems, strokes in the anterior circulation lead to expressive speech problems. In small vessel disease, the damage is largely in the subcortical and periventricular white matter. It affects those parts of the brain which contain axons connecting with the nerve cell bodies.

11.8 Do smoking and drinking affect vascular dementia?

Smoking is a major risk factor for vascular dementia, causing both large vessel and small vessel disease. Therefore all patients with a vascular dementia who smoke should be advised of this. There is no evidence to suggest that giving up smoking slows progression – this would be very difficult to prove – but common sense suggests that patients should give up smoking.

There is no problem with patients drinking a small amount of alcohol, i.e. 1–2 units/day. However, patients might be more sensitive to the effects of alcohol. Drinking large amounts of alcohol has its own effect on the brain and is also a risk factor for stroke.

11.9 What is 'Binswanger's disease'?

As in many other dementias, the naming of vascular dementia has changed over the years, which has resulted in a degree of confusion. The German pathologist Otto Binswanger was the first person to describe the arteriolosclerosis in the deep perforating arteries to the brain that results in microscopic infarcts and small vessel disease dementia. The term 'Binswanger's disease' was restricted to pathologists until the advent of CT scanning, when radiologists began to identify areas of white matter change around the ventricles; these were interpreted as small infarcts and led to the suggestion of a diagnosis of 'Binswanger's disease', which made the use of the term more widespread. However, as periventricular white matter changes are very common on CT scanning in patients with or without dementia (the changes are more marked on MRI scanning), the term 'Binswanger's disease' has fallen out of favour and is now rarely used (except by pathologists); the term 'small vessel disease' is more widely used.

11.10 How is vascular dementia diagnosed?

The clinical history and examination is crucial in the diagnosis of vascular dementia. It is important to establish whether vascular risk factors are present because it is a very unusual diagnosis in patients without risk factors. The major investigation is structural imaging with MRI or CT scanning. However, cerebral imaging can lead to overdiagnosis of vascular disease because:

■ Many individuals have asymptomatic periventricular white matter changes with increasing age. If they then develop cognitive problems for some other reason then the scan might be interpreted as showing vascular disease and a vascular dementia diagnosed.

■ Degenerative dementias, including Alzheimer's disease, are sometimes accompanied by white matter changes even in young-onset individuals. Indeed, Alzheimer's disease is often accompanied by amyloid deposition in the blood vessel walls and white matter changes – and therefore vascular changes – can play a role in the symptoms of Alzheimer's disease.

SPECT scans can be useful in diagnosing vascular dementia. In large vessel disease, SPECT scans can show multiple areas of diminished cerebral perfusion. However, this pattern is not specific and can also be seen in other individuals.

Other investigations are largely unhelpful with the exception of tests like blood cholesterol, which screen for risk factors for vascular disease.

11.11 What are the radiological features of small vessel disease?

CT and MRI scans show small vessel disease as multiple, small, discrete patches of reduced density around the ventricles (*Fig. 11.2*). These patches can coalesce in more advanced disease. Care must be taken in interpreting white matter changes on scans because:

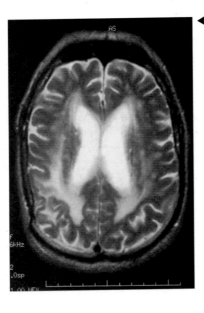

Fig. 11.2 White matter changes and focal changes from an old right parietal lobe haematoma on the MRI scan of a patient with vascular dementia.

■ white matter lesions are seen in a number of other conditions, including multiple sclerosis

■ white matter lesions are often seen in asymptomatic patients. Some of these have no vascular risk factors, others have a history of hypertension and migraine

■ different sorts of MRI brain scan have different sensitivities for showing white matter changes and some, such as FLAIR sequences, are very sensitive.

11.12 Can you distinguish vascular dementia from degenerative dementias on bedside testing or psychological tests?

The pattern of cognitive deficits in large vessel disease depends on the region of the brain affected by the strokes. In small vessel disease a more diffuse pattern is seen. Often, memory and visuospatial skills are preserved in vascular dementia unlike Alzheimer's disease. The pattern of problems in vascular dementia and frontotemporal dementia can be similar. They can both produce poor attention, poor executive skills and slow responses. Personality change is much more unusual in small vessel disease than frontotemporal dementia, insight is often preserved and tests of frontal lobe function, such as the Wisconsin Card Sorting test, are usually performed better by patients with vascular dementia than those with frontotemporal dementia.

11.13 What is the Hachinski score?

The Hachinski score is a simple scoring system that can be applied to a patient's history and examination. The scoring system is shown in *Table 11.1*. A score of less than or equal to 4 is considered to suggest a degenerative dementia, greater or equal to 7 vascular dementia.

Although the Hachinski score is quoted in virtually every textbook on dementia, it is not used clinically very often. Most of the criteria used are either self-evident – history of strokes, hemiplegias, etc. – or of debatable validity. For example, nocturnal confusion and fluctuations are typical features of dementia with Lewy bodies. However, the Hachinski score is often used in research to try to exclude cases of vascular dementia from clinical studies of Alzheimer's disease.

11.14 What is CADASIL?

CADASIL or, to give it its full name, cerebral autosomal dominant arteriopathy with subcortical ischaemic changes and leukoencephalopathy, is an inherited vascular dementia. Although only recently described it is uncommon rather than rare in neurological practice. It should be suspected in individuals who have an early onset of a vascular dementia with a history

Table 11.1 The Hachinski scoring system (© 1975 AMA with permission)

Feature	Maximum possible score
Abrupt onset	2
Stepwise deterioration	1
Fluctuating course	2
Nocturnal confusion	1
Relative preservation of personality	1
Depression	1
Somatic complaints	1
Emotional incontinence	1
History of hypertension	1
History of strokes	2
Evidence of associated atherosclerosis	1
Focal neurological symptoms	2
Focal neurological signs	2

of migraine and few vascular risk factors. Although the initial cases were described in France and the majority of cases have been reported from continental Europe, many cases have now been identified in the UK. Some patients will have a positive family history of vascular dementia, although this is often not apparent when the patient is first seen. The pattern of inheritance is autosomal dominant with high penetrance. Other family members might have been diagnosed as having atypical migraine or multiple sclerosis. The typical age for a patient to be diagnosed with CADASIL is between 35 and 55 years, although many patients have had migraine for many years prior to diagnosis. In most patients there are no clues from the migraines that they are at risk of developing a progressive vascular dementia.

The major initial investigation is an MRI scan. Once the patient has developed symptoms then the MRI brain scan is always abnormal. Indeed, the MRI scan is often abnormal prior to the onset of symptoms.

CADASIL is caused by a series of mutations in the NOTCH 3 gene on chromosome 19. The most reliable way of confirming the diagnosis is by screening for one of the series of mutations associated with the disease. Many mutations have been described and new ones continue to be discovered, so the disease can be excluded only with extensive genomic sequencing. Less direct methods of diagnosis include performing a skin biopsy and examining it for deposits in the vessel wall on electron microscopy. There is no effective treatment for CADASIL, it seems reasonable to give patients aspirin or clopidogrel if there are no contraindications.

11.15 Are there other genetic vascular dementias?

There are other rare vascular dementias. One is called Fabry's disease, which is a combination of strokes, painful sensory symptoms and a rash. There are also many genetic conditions that predispose to stroke, including some forms of diabetes, high lipids in the blood, homocysteinuria, etc. Patients with these conditions will be predisposed to develop a vascular dementia.

11.16 What are the risk factors for vascular disease?

- Hypertension.
- Hypercholesterolaemia.
- Diabetes.
- Polycythaemia.
- Male sex.
- Racial, e.g. of African–Caribbean extraction.
- Valvular heart disease.
- Atrial fibrillation.
- Smoking.
- Age.
- Family history.
- Other vascular disease – ischaemic heart disease, peripheral vascular disease.
- Polycythaemia – too many red cells.
- Renal disease.

11.17 Do patients with vascular dementia need to be referred to a neurologist?

It is unusual for patients with multi-infarct dementia to be referred to a neurology outpatient department. Very often the diagnosis is clear and the physical handicaps from the strokes so dominate the clinical picture that there seems little point in referring to a neurologist. In the early stages of the disease, referral to a neurologist, cardiologist or physician is important to exclude a cause for recurrent stroke, such as paroxysmal atrial fibrillation.

Small vessel disease is more difficult to diagnose and investigations can be harder to interpret. Patients with small vessel disease might well be referred to a neurologist.

11.18 What physical signs suggest a diagnosis of multi-infarct dementia?

The presence of physical signs is a pointer to multi-infarct dementia, although more weight should be put on the history than the examination.

Sudden events, often with some improvement over days, suggest a vascular dementia; a more gradual onset suggests a space-occupying lesion or degenerative disease.

The typical physical signs accompanying vascular dementia include hemiplegia, dysphasia and hemianopia. There might be physical signs to suggest a source of emboli causing the dementia, such as an irregularly irregular pulse or mitral stenotic murmur.

11.19 What investigations are needed in multi-infarct dementia?

Investigations should have two aims: the diagnosis of the dementia and the search for treatable risk factors to reduce the chance of further strokes. The first part is addressed in Chapter 1. If there is doubt about the diagnosis, patients should have cranial imaging. Investigations to look for the cause of the strokes should include:

- full blood count
- urea and electrolytes
- cholesterol and lipids
- blood glucose
- chest X-ray
- electrocardiogram
- erythrocyte sedimentation rate or equivalent
- syphilis serology.

Many more specialist investigations might be needed in patients with a rapidly progressive history or other unusual features. These can be aimed at the heart:

- 24-hour rhythm electrocardiograms
- transthoracic or transoesophageal echocardiograms

or at looking for a vasculitis:

- lupus screen, including anticardiolipin antibodies and lupus anticoagulant
- other autoantibodies
- examination of urinary sediment for casts
- cerebral angiography.

11.20 How is vascular dementia treated?

There is no convincing evidence that the cholinesterase inhibitors are effective in vascular dementia, although a couple of very small studies suggest a possible benefit. A number of treatments should be considered (*Box 11.1*). There are few treatment trials for vascular dementia and therefore the advice in the box is based on the guidance in prevention of strokes.

Box 11.1 Treatments for vascular dementia

Antihypertensive:

Give if the blood pressure is raised. The threshold for treatment will vary with the clinical features. Evidence is accumulating to suggest that lowering blood pressure, even when it is within the 'physiological range', will reduce the chance of further strokes in stroke patients. Until recently the choice of antihypertensive was unclear but recent evidence suggests that patients with a clinical stroke will benefit from a combination of an ACE (angiotensin-converting enzyme) inhibitor such as perindopril and a thiazide such as Xapamide.

Statin:

Until recently the normal range for cholesterol was up to 6.9 mmol/L and only levels above this would be treated. Now, following trials in patients with cardiovascular disease, patients with a clinical stroke are being treated with a statin if their cholesterol is greater than 5.0 mmol/L. It is also becoming common to prescribe statins regardless of the baseline cholesterol because the most recent evidence suggests that the substantial reduction of cholesterol levels seen with statins reduces the risk of further stroke even in patients who start with low cholesterol levels.

Aspirin or clopidogrel:

There is good evidence that aspirin or clopidogrel reduces the risk of a stroke by about 20% in individuals with vascular disease. Both these drugs can therefore be considered in patients with a vascular dementia, providing they do not have coexistent disease that precludes either drug. The choice between the two is evenly balanced. There is very wide experience of aspirin and it has been shown to be effective in a wide range of vascular problems; clopidogrel might be slightly superior in efficacy but is much less tested. The usual dose of aspirin is 75 or 150 mg per day. Higher doses have a higher complication rate without clear additional benefit. The dose of clopidogrel is 75 mg daily. Clopidogrel should be used in patients unable to tolerate aspirin.

The drugs should be used with common sense. A patient with a severe dementia will obtain little benefit from these treatments and they should be used sparingly. A hypertensive, hypercholesterolaemic patient with a clinical history of stroke plus a mild vascular dementia and good quality of life could be given quadruple treatment – a statin, aspirin, an ACE inhibitor and a thiazide.

Other medical conditions predisposing to stroke, such as diabetes and valvular heart disease, will need specific treatment.

11.21 What is the prognosis of vascular dementia?

Despite the advent of a number of treatments, the prognosis of vascular dementia is similar to that of Alzheimer's disease – the disease tends to be progressive with death on average 7 years after diagnosis. Patients who are treated for a specific cause, such as valvular heart disease, might have a better prognosis.

11.22 How can the gait problems in small vessel disease be helped?

Unfortunately, very little can be done to alleviate the typical gait problems seen in small vessel disease – the so-called apraxic gait. The problem is with the central planning of movement. Aids to help a patient rise from a chair, a stick and encouragement at the onset of walking can be helpful. Physiotherapists can give advice and occupational therapists help with suitable aids.

11.23 What is the future of vascular dementia?

There seems little doubt that vascular dementia will continue to be a major health problem. In the immediate future it seems likely that any blood pressure and/or cholesterol level that is 'too high', and any patient presenting with a stroke, will be started on quadruple therapy of a statin, an antiplatelet drug (usually aspirin), a thiazide and an ACE inhibitor.

More invasive techniques and higher medical priority for the prevention and acute treatment of stroke might reduce the incidence of vascular dementia.

PATIENT QUESTIONS

11.24 What lifestyle changes help prevent deterioration in vascular dementia?

There is little direct evidence that lifestyle changes can help vascular dementia but it is sensible to follow the advice given to patients who have had strokes or who have Alzheimer's disease:

- exercise is good: a daily walk for 20–30 minutes is sufficient but a bit more is ideal
- keep your mind active with conversation, crosswords, reading, etc.
- eat a diet that is low in saturated fat and low in cholesterol
- lose weight if you are over your ideal weight (body mass index greater than 25)
- give up smoking
- avoid excess alcohol (more than 2 units/day): a glass of red wine a day might help
- talk to your GP about taking aspirin
- if you have diabetes, control it carefully
- have your blood pressure checked regularly – annually if it is normal; every 3 months if it is raised.

11.25 My husband has vascular dementia. Are my children at risk too?

The vast majority of cases of vascular dementia are not the result of genetic diseases and therefore the risk of passing them on to children is small. However, very rare forms of vascular dementia are inherited. The most common is CADASIL (*see Q 11.13*). Many of the inherited vascular dementias described in the old literature were cases of CADASIL. Many of the risk factors for vascular dementia do run in families – hypertension, obesity, high cholesterol – and it is sensible to advise your children to treat their risk factors (*see Q 11.23*).

Frontotemporal dementia

12

12.1 What is frontotemporal dementia?

Frontotemporal dementia (FTD) is one of the common forms of degenerative dementia. It is less familiar to GPs and physicians than other forms of degenerative dementia, partly because it has undergone a series of changes of name in the last 30 years but also because there are many different subtypes. The frontal lobes are the large lobes at the front of the brain; the temporal lobes are situated laterally on each side of the brain. Together they account for over half the brain. It is therefore not surprising that there are a number of variants of FTD (*Fig. 12.1*). 'Frontotemporal dementia' is a broad term and the following are either old names for types of FTD or varieties of FTD:

- Pick's disease
- frontal lobe degeneration of non-Alzheimer type
- dementia lacking distinctive pathology
- semantic dementia
- frontal lobe dementia/dementia of frontal type
- primary progressive aphasia/primary non-fluent aphasia
- motor neuron disease dementia
- right temporal lobe atrophy.

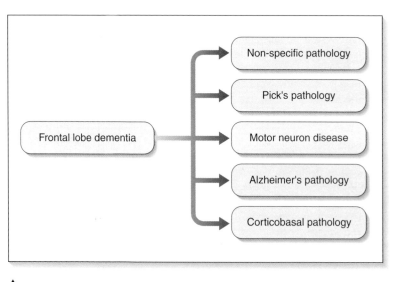

▲

Fig. 12.1 Clinical frontotemporal dementia can be produced by a number of different pathological processes.

12.2 How does FTD differ from Alzheimer's disease?

> Although the outlook for carers and patients is similar in some ways to Alzheimer's disease, there are a number of important differences:
>
> ■ behavioural problems are an early troublesome feature
> ■ the patient loses insight and undergoes personality changes – these are both very distressing for partners; personality change is a late feature in Alzheimer's disease, and indeed might never occur
> ■ memory is often preserved
> ■ there is a higher incidence of familial cases.

12.3 What is Pick's disease?

Pick's disease is an old name for FTD. Arnold Pick was a German psychiatrist who described the problems experienced by four patients who had lost brain tissue in their frontal or temporal lobes. In many ways it would have been simpler to copy the example of Alzheimer's disease and describe all patients presenting with an FTD as having Pick's disease. However, this is not possible because the term 'Pick's disease' was used very widely in the twentieth century to refer to many different diseases. As a result, it has become impossible to define what the term now actually means and most clinicians feel that it is too confusing to be kept in use.

Having said this, the term 'Pick's disease' *is* still used sometimes – mainly as a result of old habits dying hard but some neurologists and psychiatrists use it for a small proportion of patients with FTD who have severe atrophy of the frontal and temporal lobes. Pathologists (who live in a more definite world) also use the term – for patients with well-defined, knife-edge atrophy of the frontal and temporal lobes (*Figs 12.2 and 12.3*) and the distinctive inclusion bodies and cells described by Alzheimer (just to confuse matters further) in one of the early cases of Pick's disease.

12.4 How common is FTD?

FTD is mainly a presenile dementia. It is about equally common in men and women. There are few epidemiologically sound measures of its frequency and most estimates compare its frequency with that of Alzheimer's disease. FTD is relatively uncommon in the elderly population compared with Alzheimer's disease. Therefore most GPs and care-of-the-elderly psychiatrists and physicians see few cases. Clinicians who deal with younger patients see it much more commonly and it is not uncommon in specialized memory clinics. This is probably because of bias – patients with

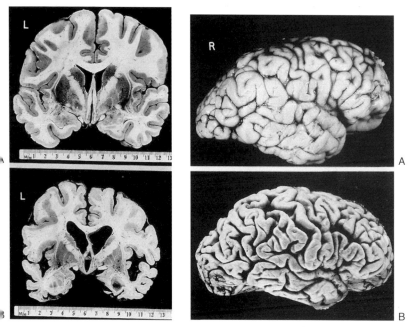

Fig. 12.2 A coronal section of the brain in frontotemporal dementia is shown in the lower part of the figure. The upper part shows a normal brain for comparison.

Fig. 12.3 External appearance of the brain in frontotemporal dementia. The upper part shows a normal brain. The lower part shows the brain of a patient with frontotemporal dementia showing atrophy of the temporal pole.

the striking features of FTD are more likely to be referred to a tertiary centre than patients with Alzheimer's disease. In memory clinics, 10% or more of patients with a presenile dementia have FTD.

12.5 What is the cause of sporadic FTD?

This remains an almost complete mystery. Genetic factors play a role in many cases but there must also be environmental triggers, the nature of which is unknown.

TYPES OF FTD

12.6 Are there different types of FTD?

Yes, unlike Alzheimer's disease, which can have a varied presentation but is essentially a single disease, FTD is probably a series of diseases with the common feature of selectively affecting the frontal and temporal lobes. These lobes account for much of the cerebral cortex – the 'thinking part' of the brain – and therefore the term 'frontotemporal dementia' is less discriminating than one might think.

12.7 What are the different types of FTD?

The description of different types of FTD is complicated because FTD can be subdivided in a number of different ways. In the clinic there are three common types:

■ Dementia of frontal type: patients develop behavioural and emotional problems. It is associated with frontal lobe atrophy.
■ Primary progressive aphasia (PPA): patients develop a slowly progressive difficulty in language that shows itself with difficulty finding the right word and later in reading and writing. PPA has recently been renamed 'progressive non-fluent aphasia', which is a more accurate term but the older term is still widely used in clinical practice. It is associated with dominant perisylvian atrophy.
■ Semantic dementia: patients lose their knowledge of the meaning of words. This tends to present as progressive fluent aphasia. It is associated with dominant anterior temporal lobe atrophy.

12.8 What is dementia of the frontal type?

This is the typical FTD; clinicians often use the terms 'frontotemporal dementia' and 'dementia of frontal type' interchangeably. Typically, patients start with an emotional or behavioural change. The most common behavioural changes are apathy and disinhibition:

■ Apathetic patients lose interest in family and hobbies and gradually do less and less. However, there are many other causes of apathy, for example depression.
■ Disinhibition is the loss of the usual inhibitions. These can be relatively mild, for example starting to talk to strangers or picking up other people's used glasses in a public house, or extreme – walking around with a cardboard box on their head.

Certain types of behavioural change cause particular problems:

■ Overspending: this is often subtle and secretive at first and the patient's spouse can be aghast when a credit card bill for £5000 arrives. The money might be spent on the similar items again and again. One patient bought 150 similar jumpers from Marks and Spencer.
■ Lack of hygiene: a common problem is giving up washing or not washing clothes. Patients often lose pride in their personal appearance.

- ■ 'Criminal' behaviour: a common problem is 'shop lifting'. The patient starts taking items from shops without paying for them. This behavioural problem can normally be easily distinguished from the criminal kind by the lack of any attempt to hide the items. The person just picks up a pack of their favourite sweets and walks out with it. Occasionally individuals are prosecuted, sometimes repeatedly.

- ■ Sexual behaviour: this is particularly distressing for spouses and it needs to be stressed repeatedly to relatives that the behaviour stems from the disease and not from the person. This can involve children or other forms of abnormal sexuality. Fortunately, talking about sex and viewing pornography is more common than any action – indeed spouses often comment that libido is reduced. Nevertheless, even talking about sex to children is a serious matter and if there is any hint of this kind of problem then precautions are essential.

- ■ Eating behaviour: eating habits often change. Patients change their food preference and start eating more sweet food. Eating habits change and table manners deteriorate, with food often being stuffed into the mouth. Some sufferers will eat all the food they can see, others will actively seek food and eat it. In extreme forms, patients put non-food items in their mouth. Smoking and drinking alcohol can also increase early in the illness, presumably due to a similar mechanism.

- ■ Stereotyped behaviours: this is the repeated performance of an action. It can be simple, such as checking that a door is closed or repeatedly washing hands, but many patients have more complex stereotypes. A common one is a stereotyped walk, often several miles long, during which the patient takes exactly the same route at the same time. These behaviours can be misdiagnosed as an obsessive–compulsive disorder.

Emotional change is often more subtle but distressing. The person might show no emotional response at the funeral of a parent or become very 'cold' to a loved partner.

12.9 What is a typical story of a patient with dementia of the frontal type?

CASE STUDY

Anna Sandringham is a 62-year-old farmer. Her husband noted that she was becoming less affectionate to him and her grandchildren. She gradually withdrew from the work on the farm and began to sit in the house watching television. She started to go to church again and began to go to every service. She would set off for church 40 minutes before the service and follow the same roundabout route every day, calling in at the same newsagent each day but never buying anything. She had been a keen chess player and continued to play to her previous high standard except that she began to cheat occasionally. She needed persuasion to wash and her husband had to take over the washing of her clothes.

12.10 Primary progressive aphasia/progressive non-fluent aphasia

Primary progressive aphasia is very different from the other forms of FTD. The patient's problems are at first limited to the production of words in speech, usually beginning with word-finding difficulty although some forms start with pure difficulty in the production of sound. The problems progress and when reading and writing are also affected it becomes clear that the primary problem is one of language. The problems typically remain limited to language for a long period – often for years. Some patients then develop typical behavioural problems suggestive of FTD; these patients usually have the pathological changes characteristic of FTD. Other patients later develop more widespread cognitive problems – usually related to memory and route-finding – which are reminiscent of Alzheimer's disease, and indeed the pathological changes in many patients are those of Alzheimer's disease.

12.11 What is a typical story of a patient with primary progressive aphasia?

CASE STUDY

Sydney Wells is a 62-year-old ironmonger. He started to have difficulty remembering the names of certain items he sold. At first the difficulty was apparent only to himself and his assistant, because customers would normally ask for what they wanted and Sydney would not need to say the name. However, as his problems worsened he started to have problems with telephone conversations and with complex discussions. His word-finding difficulties became apparent in day-to-day conversation, he had difficulty in writing down telephone messages on the pad by the phone and he gave up reading. For 2 years his problems remained those of language but then his assistant complained that he was no longer doing his share of the work in the shop. He would stand by the phone and ignore customers, especially those he failed to recognize, and he no longer cared for the shop or for his personal appearance in the way that he had.

12.12 What is semantic dementia?

Semantic dementia is a rare form of FTD in which patients lose their memory for facts. Although semantic dementia has only recently been recognized as a form of dementia, descriptions of the condition appear in the older literature, albeit under different names, so it is not a new disease.

In semantic dementia, common words no longer mean anything to the patient. To everyone else the word 'goat' conjures-up a picture of a four-legged animal with a beard; to a patient with semantic dementia the word 'goat' may have no more meaning than a nonsense word like 'geat'. Patients find it difficult to find the right word for objects but, unlike other patients with naming problems resulting from different causes, they cannot give information about the object either. For example, patients with various neurological problems might have difficulty in naming a picture of a giraffe. But if asked to point to the animal with a long neck that lived in Africa they would do so. Patients with semantic dementia have lost the meaning behind the word 'giraffe' and are therefore not helped by such clues.

By contrast, the autobiographical memory of patients with FTD is usually well preserved and they can recall events of the previous day. Imaging typically shows selective left temporal lobe atrophy (*Fig. 12.4*) or bilateral temporal lobe atrophy.

As the disease progresses, the person develops other problems similar to those seen in other forms of FTD, with changes in emotion and behaviour.

12.13 What is a typical story of a patient with semantic dementia?

CASE STUDY

Joy Dersingham is a 58-year-old banker. She was reading at her desk one day when a colleague asked her to pass the stapler. 'What is a stapler?' she replied. This was initially excused as a joke but, increasingly, her colleagues and husband noticed that she was having difficulty in finding the right word for objects and would lose the meaning of everyday words. Her problems progressed. Then, when asked to read the lesson in church, she mispronounced the names of several prophets and this prompted her husband to seek medical advice. Her problems progressed and she began to speak less. She gained weight because she began to eat sweet foods excessively and she started to spend money recklessly.

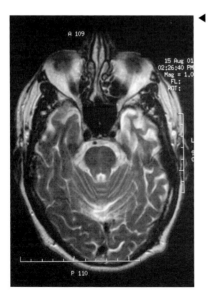

Fig. 12.4 MRI scan showing selective left temporal pole atrophy in a patient with semantic dementia.

ASSESSING AND HELPING PATIENTS WITH FTD

12.14 How good is the MMSE at assessing patients with FTD?

The MMSE was designed with Alzheimer's disease in mind and tends to test those parts of cognition that are affected early in Alzheimer's disease. Patients with FTD can therefore score very well on the MMSE and, in a couple of cases, patients who were very disabled with FTD scored full marks (30/30) on the MMSE. The test cannot, therefore, be used to screen for FTD.

When doing the MMSE, the first abnormalities displayed by patients with FTD are rather variable. Often, patients will behave in an abnormal way when doing the test. In the three-part command they will perseverate with folding the piece of paper until they can fold it no more, or, when asked to write a sentence, they will write an inappropriate word or phrase. Patients often will not pay attention or make an effort with the tests, which again produces variable results. Orientation to time goes before orientation to place, some patients find the serial 7s difficult. Copying the pentagons is usually preserved, unless patients perseverate or decide to do their own, alternative drawing, as shown in *Fig. 12.5* – when asked to copy a pentagon this patient refused and instead persevered in writing 'nil wilton'.

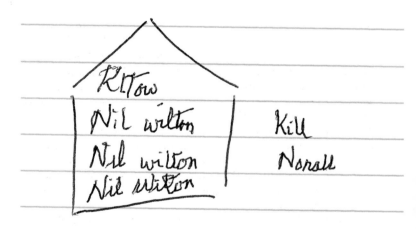

▲

Fig. 12.5 The patient was asked to copy the pentagon. He did not, but instead persevered in writing 'Nil Wilton' and 'Kill Nonall' in an aggressive manner.

Box 12.1 Tests used to detect frontal lobe problems

Proverb interpretation:

To test proverb interpretation the patient is asked the meaning of well-known phrases such as 'Too many cooks spoil the broth' or 'A stitch in time saves nine'. Allowances are made for the intellectual and cultural background of the patient. Patients with FTD tend to give concrete answers – essentially repeating back the phrase to the examiner – 'Well, if you have too many cooks the broth will be spoilt'.

Cognitive estimates:

To test cognitive estimates the patient is asked to estimate numerical values for quantities such as:

- the height of a well known building, e.g. Canary Wharf
- how fast a horse gallops
- how many miles is it to London from Norwich

Patients with FTD tend to estimate poorly. They might say a horse gallops at 10 mph. In borderline cases, patients are given the chance to adjust their answer by the examiner asking 'Is that too slow or too fast'. FTD patients fail to correct when given the chance.

12.15 What simple tests can I do to test frontal lobe function?

Two of the more common bedside tests used to detect frontal lobe problems are the interpretation of proverbs and cognitive estimates (patients estimate numerical values for unknown quantities) (*Box 12.1*).

12.16 What physical signs are found in FTD?

The majority of patients with FTD will have no physical signs on examination. Some have release reflexes (*see Q 2.44*) early in the course of the disease. Other signs, such as a field defect or lack of sense of smell, suggest that the patient's problems are caused by a tumour. Rare forms of FTD can develop prominent features of Parkinson's disease early in the course of the illness. Late in the disease, patients with FTD might have more marked physical signs suggesting pyramidal and extrapyramidal disease.

A minority of patients with FTD who have motor neuron disease dementia often show signs of motor neuron disease:

- spastic dysarthria
- wasted fasiculating tongue

- weakness of neck muscles
- wasted weak limbs
- brisk tendon reflexes.

12.17 Do patients with FTD realize they are ill?

It is characteristic of FTD that patients are either totally unaware that they have a dementia or have only a very limited insight into their problems.

12.18 What treatments are available for FTD?

Non-drug treatments for FTD are discussed in Chapter 5. The drug treatment of FTD remains disappointing. Unfortunately, no drugs have been shown to improve or change the natural history of FTD. FTD is rare and currently drugs aimed specifically at FTD are unlikely to be developed. Advances in treatment depend on further advances aimed at understanding the pathogenesis of the disease or the development of treatments for related conditions such as Alzheimer's disease. The cholinesterase inhibitors, such as rivastigmine or galantamine, might improve the symptoms, but this has not yet been established.

 Drug treatments are used for behavioural problems. Traditionally, the drugs used were neuroleptics, such as haloperidol or sulpiride. However, these can cause severe extrapyramidal side-effects and the newer antipsychotics, such as risperidone or olanzapine, are now used. These are discussed in more detail on page 92. Occasionally, other sedative drugs are used. Some of the behavioural problems, such as overeating and stereotyped routines, are now being treated successfully with specific serotonin reuptake inhibitors (SSRIs); this is not a licensed indication for these drugs.

12.19 Can patients with FTD drive?

Driving is a particular problem with FTD. Indeed, road traffic accidents can be the reason for referral to a specialist. Patients with FTD can lack the judgement necessary to drive and, furthermore, do not care about this and lack insight into their problems. This makes them particularly dangerous drivers. Often, forceful methods such as selling the car are necessary to stop FTD patients driving. There are exceptions, and patients with an isolated progressive aphasia might drive perfectly competently. Driving is also discussed in Chapter 7.

12.20 What typical abnormalities are seen in neuropsychological testing in FTD?

Frontal lobe problems lead to problems with attention and in the planning and execution of tasks. Patients do poorly in several neuropsychological tests:

■ The Wisconsin Card Sorting test: patients are required to sort cards into different groups according to different criteria – colour, shape, etc. The patients are given cards not unlike playing cards with different symbols of different shapes and colours. They are asked to sort the cards by a self-chosen category and told if they are correct. Then the examiner changes the rules and the patients need to learn to sort by a different category. Patients with FTD often start well but perseverate in the categories – failing to learn the new rules and going back to the old ones.

■ The Stroop test: this test comprises a chart containing a list of the names of colours printed in other colours – so the word 'red' might be printed in blue ink. Patients have to read the list according to the colour of the ink not the word – inhibiting the dominant response. Patients with FTD have great difficulty doing this.

■ The Tower of London test: patients have to plan movements of coloured beads to achieve a certain pattern. Patients are asked to move a bead from one stand to another but to do so according to a set of rules and by moving other beads first. Patients with FTD have difficulty planning such tasks.

Temporal lobe tests include tests of semantic memory. Patients with a semantic dementia do poorly on:

■ Naming line drawings.
■ The pronunciation of irregularly spelt words, such as soot, dough and pint. Patients do not recognize the words and pronounce them according to the common grammatical rules.
■ The pyramids and palm trees test: patients must match objects according to a link between them. Patients are asked to link a picture of one object with one of two alternatives. In the classic example patients are given a picture of pyramid and asked to link it either with a picture of fir trees or one of palm trees. Semantic knowledge tells us that the pyramid is linked to the palm trees but patients with semantic dementia are as likely to link the pyramid with the fir trees as with the palm trees.

Patients with progressive aphasia do poorly on confrontational naming and in spontaneous speech, for example in the Boston Cookie test when they have to describe the events shown in a picture. Some have difficulty with the repetition of digits in the Digit Span test or with the repetition of words or phrases.

12.21 What investigations are useful in FTD?

Although it is very unusual for a patient with a typical story for Alzheimer's disease to have a tumour, tumours can mimic FTD. A CT or MRI scan should therefore be considered in all FTD patients. Typical appearances of diffuse frontal atrophy are shown in *Fig. 12.6*. If structural imaging is normal then functional imaging such as PET scanning or SPECT might show abnormalities (see Chapter 2). Other investigations are similar to those for Alzheimer's disease. An EEG is sometimes useful in the diagnosis of FTD; it is characteristically normal early in the disease whereas a patient with Alzheimer's disease of a similar severity will show slowing of the dominant rhythm.

12.22 Is there a society for patients with FTD?

There is no exact equivalent of the Alzheimer's Society (www.alzheimers.org.uk) but the Alzheimer's Society does provide information on FTD; the organization Counselling and Diagnosis in Dementia (CANDID; www.candid.ion.ucl.ac.uk) can also help. There are also a number of local support groups.

12.23 Is FTD inherited?

FTD is usually a sporadic disease affecting only one person in a family. However, familial forms are well known and a positive family history for dementia is more common in FTD than in Alzheimer's disease. The best estimates are that about 1 in 5 affected individuals has a parent or sibling with the disease. A few large pedigrees are known in which patients might develop FTD. One such family tree is shown in *Fig. 12.7*.

12.24 What genetic defects can cause FTD?

The genetic cause for about 15% of familial FTD has been discovered. These individuals have mutations in the microtubule-associated protein gene called tau, which lies on chromosome 17. Many different mutations have been described and some are more common than others. Individuals with tau mutations can have typical FTD or might have more prominent parkinsonian and other extrapyramidal problems than typical FTD.

There is also evidence that genes on chromosome 3 and chromosome 9 can cause FTD; it is quite possible that more genes await discovery.

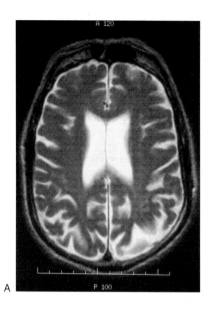

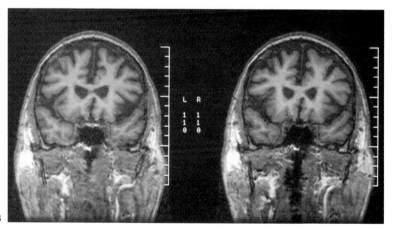

Fig. 12.6 A. Diffuse frontal lobe atrophy seen on an MRI scan in a patient with frontotemporal dementia. B. This is seen more clearly on coronal sections from the same scan.

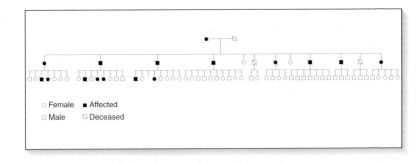

▲

Fig. 12.7 Pedigree with autosomal dominant frontotemporal dementia. Eight of the original 12 children developed frontotemporal dementia.

12.25 Can individuals be screened for tau mutations?

At the moment this isn't possible. The mutations are too rare and too many in number to allow general screening. However, such screening will almost certainly become available in time. Individuals at high risk of having a tau mutation, for example someone affected with FTD plus parkinsonism whose mother and grandmother had a similar disease, can often help with research projects and might be offered screening for tau mutations by research groups.

12.26 What are the particular problems of dealing with patients with FTD?

The particular problems of FTD are caused by the personality and behavioural changes. These are distressing for relatives, particularly if the behaviour is of a violent or sexual type. Most patients with Alzheimer's disease remain recognizable as the person they are. Many patients with FTD become new people to their spouses and behave in way they would never have done before they became ill.

12.27 Can the hyperphagia be treated?

Hyperphagia can be a particular problem, the patient might gain excessive weight or their eating habits can be embarrassing. Sometimes, simple modifications to the environment can make a large difference. Many patients with hyperphagia will not actively seek out food (although some do) but only eat what they can see. Smaller portions and keeping serving plates out of sight can help. Drug treatment with SSRIs can be beneficial

12.28 What is the prognosis of FTD?

The prognosis overall is similar to Alzheimer's disease, with average life expectancy about 7 years from diagnosis. Like Alzheimer's disease, rapidly progressive cases are unusual and those that do occur often are in association with motor neuron disease. Patients with a purely frontal syndrome might have a very prolonged course and can be little changed from year to year.

12.29 What is the future of FTD?

There have been major advances in the understanding of the genetics of FTD. One gene has been located on chromosome 17 and has been shown to be the gene coding for the microtubule-associated protein tau. Other genes are linked to the short arm of chromosome 3 and possibly chromosome 9. Hopefully, further research will lead to a clear understanding of the pathogenesis of FTD and allow the development of drugs targeted at specific sites in the pathological cascade.

In the more immediate future, the cholinesterase inhibitors might prove effective in FTD.

 PATIENT QUESTIONS

12.30 What do the frontal lobes do?

Our knowledge of frontal lobe function is not complete. The most posterior part of the frontal lobes is the so-called 'motor strip'. This is the area that sends impulses via the brainstem and spinal cord to move our muscles. Damage to the motor strip causes paralysis of the opposite side of the body; this can be partial or complete. An area just forward of this is an important speech area called Broca's area. Damage to this causes difficulty in the production of speech. The areas further forward of these regions are harder to investigate. We know from studies of individuals who have had bullet wounds, strokes or other problems involving the front of the frontal lobes that they regulate and plan our behaviour. They are also responsible for many of the characteristics that make up our personality.

12.31 What do the temporal lobes do?

The most medial (middle) part of the temporal lobe is concerned with recent memory and is typically involved in Alzheimer's disease. Memories that are related to facts are stored more laterally, in the so-called 'semantic memory'. This area also helps us recognize faces. The parts of the temporal lobes furthest forward are concerned with emotion, smell, eating behaviour and personality.

12.32 What symptoms suggest an FTD?

Typical FTD starts with one of three problems:

- Personality change: the person can either become apathetic and withdrawn, showing little interest in hobbies, or more extrovert and start talking to strangers. Patients who become apathetic and withdrawn are often initially thought to be depressed.
- Behavioural change: the person develops new behaviours. These can be the result of disinhibition, common examples include swearing in public or overspending. Another form of behavioural change is the development of stereotyped behaviours. In some patients these behaviours have a religious flavour.
- Emotional change: the person shows no concern for friends or family and exhibits no empathy with others.

12.33 What are the chances of treatments becoming available for FTDs?

In the immediate future, we should soon know whether the cholinesterase inhibitors are effective in FTD.

The long-term goal of a more effective treatment is likely to occur as a result of genetic discoveries giving us more clues to the cause of FTD.

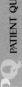

PATIENT QUESTIONS

Parkinson's disease, Huntington's disease and dementia

13

DEMENTIA AND PARKINSON'S DISEASE

DEMENTIA AND PARKINSON'S DISEASE

13.1 What is the difference between Parkinson's disease and parkinsonism?

Parkinson's disease is a common disorder that affects approximately 1 in 100 individuals by the age of 70 years. It was originally described – very accurately – by James Parkinson, a nineteenth-century physician, and is named after him. It is important to distinguish Parkinson's disease (sometimes called idiopathic Parkinson's disease) from parkinsonism. Parkinson's disease is a distinct disease that has a classical clinical triad of tremor, bradykinesia and rigidity. It is caused by death of dopaminergic nerve cells projecting to the substantia nigra. Parkinsonism describes conditions other than Parkinson's disease that mimic Parkinson's disease. There are many causes of parkinsonism, the most common is neuroleptic drugs but a number of diseases including cerebrovascular disease, progressive supranuclear palsy and corticobasal degeneration can exhibit some other features of Parkinson's disease.

Subtle differences between the clinical features of Parkinson's disease and parkinsonism allow the clinician to distinguish them in most patients. Inevitably, however, some patients fall between the two categories and sometimes time is needed to distinguish Parkinson's disease and parkinsonism. There are many distinctions but two of the most useful are the typical, coarse Parkinson's disease tremor, which is unusual in parkinsonism, and the disappointing response of parkinsonism to treatment with L-dopa.

When the brainstem of patients with idiopathic Parkinson's disease is examined a distinctive inclusion – the Lewy body – is seen. This is the cardinal pathological feature of Parkinson's disease.

The relationship between the various parkinsonian syndromes and dementia is discussed in Chapter 14.

13.2 Is Parkinson's disease associated with memory problems?

Although James Parkinson described all the motor features of his disease, he did not recognize the associated cognitive problems and for many years it was felt that memory problems were rare in Parkinson's disease. This view has now changed and it is accepted that most patients with Parkinson's disease have minor cognitive abnormalities on formal memory testing. These problems do not usually concern the patient. Unfortunately, some of these patients later develop a dementia.

In some patients, cognitive problems precede the development of the typical motor problems of Parkinson's disease. In the last

15 years there has been an explosion of interest in these patients with a combination of parkinsonism and memory problems. Many of these patients have Lewy bodies in the cerebral cortex as well as the brainstem, and also have some of the pathological changes of Alzheimer's disease. Various names have been used to describe such patients but a consensus statement in 1998 decided on the name 'dementia with Lewy bodies' (DLB).

13.3 What is the difference between Parkinson's disease with dementia and dementia with Lewy bodies (DLB)?

The same group of clinicians and pathologists who decided upon the name 'dementia with Lewy bodies' (DLB) also divided patients with cognitive problems and Parkinson's disease into two groups: patients with early cognitive problems were described as having DLB and individuals who had the motor features of Parkinson's disease for over a year before developing cognitive problems were said to have 'Parkinson's disease with dementia'. This distinction is rather artificial because, clinically and pathologically, the two diseases are on a spectrum.

The two ends of the spectrum are distinct. Patients who, after several years of purely motor problems, develop some mild slowing of thought, apathy and forgetfulness are typical of Parkinson's disease with dementia. Patients with a rapidly progressive dementia with fluctuations, hallucinations, myoclonus but only mild parkinsonian features have DLB. Many patients fall between these two extremes.

In this chapter, the term 'dementia with Lewy bodies/Parkinson's dementia' (DLB/PD) will be used to refer to features common to the two diseases.

13.4 What are Lewy bodies?

Lewy bodies are small intracellular inclusion bodies. They can be round or oval shaped and have a distinct halo. They are eosinophilic on haematoxylin and eosin (H&E) staining. In the brainstem they are easy to pick out on H&E stains and have long been recognized as the pathological hallmark of Parkinson's disease. In the cerebral cortex they are less easy to see on H&E stains but modern anti-ubiquitin stains make them easy to see and count. One of the major reasons for the increase in interest and recognition of DLB has been the ease with which Lewy bodies can now be detected in the cortex. Recently, the use of alpha-synuclein stains has led to further improvements in Lewy body detection.

13.5 What are the clinical motor features of Parkinson's disease?

Parkinson's disease generally presents with a tremor in one hand, which is most prominent when the arm is at rest. The tremor is rather coarse and of slower frequency than the typical essential tremor. Many patients' tremor includes some pronation and supination, with a movement of the thumb over the forefinger leading to the description of a pill-rolling tremor. As the disease progresses, the hand becomes stiff and slow. The earliest sign of this is often seen in the handwriting which becomes smaller – micrographia. Typically, the micrographia is progressive and the writing becomes smaller towards the end of a sentence. The disease tends to spread slowly to involve the leg on the same side, then the contralateral arm and finally the contralateral leg. The patient's gait slows down with reduced arm swing and becomes more stooped. Many patients tend to dribble (sialorrhoea) and their speech becomes quieter and a little slurred.

The stiffness and slowness (rigidity and bradykinesia) of Parkinson's disease can be improved by drugs, which boost the dopaminergic function in the cells of the brainstem. The tremor also responds, but less reliably. The response to treatment is so reliable that it is part of the diagnosis. Lack of response to L-dopa or similar drugs suggest that the patient has parkinsonism rather than Parkinson's disease.

13.6 Are there criteria for diagnosing DLB?

Yes, an international consortium has produced guidelines for the diagnosis (McKeith et al 1996). These are summarized below:

- The patient must have a progressive dementia.
- The patient must have two of the following three features:
  - marked fluctuations in cognition; these can be within one day or day to day
  - persistent, well-formed visual hallucinations
  - spontaneous parkinsonism.
- The following features are supportive:
  - recurrent falls
  - syncope
  - neuroleptic sensitivity
  - systemized delusions
  - non-visual hallucinations.

13.7 What are the typical features of the memory problems seen in DLB or DLB/PD?

The common cognitive problems of Parkinson's disease and dementia with Lewy bodies fall into three groups:

■ Difficulty in planning tasks: this is called executive function and can manifest as apathy.

■ A general slowness in thought and response: slowness of motor movements can disguise the cognitive problems or accentuate them.

■ Visual hallucinations: these are made worse by dopaminergic drugs but they can occur spontaneously. When they occur without other cognitive problems they do not necessarily mean that the patient will develop a dementia. The common visual hallucinations are of figures or animals. The figures might be people the patient recognizes or faceless individuals; they might appear as angels or other mythical beings. The hallucinations can be very persistent – sometimes a daily occurrence.

One of the characteristic features of DLB is fluctuation in the cognitive symptoms. These can be very dramatic and sometimes result in hospitalization in an 'acute confusional state' for which no cause is found. Some individuals have fluctuations over short periods of time – hours – whereas others fluctuate over days.

13.8 How common is DLB?

Groups with an interest in DLB suggest that it accounts for 15–25% of all cases of degenerative dementia who have postmortem examinations. These figures demonstrate that DLB is a common degenerative dementia but the collection of patients by such groups introduces a number of biases and therefore these figures are no more than a guide to its prevalence in the community. Similarly, patients with DLB account for a significant proportion of patients with dementia seen in memory clinics because the psychiatric and neurological problems associated with DLB often result in early tertiary referral to such clinics. True epidemiological data is hard to collect because the diagnosis is only made for certain at postmortem.

13.9 Do patients with DLB/PD have non-visual hallucinations?

The hallucinations of DLB/PD are most commonly visual but many patients also have other forms of hallucination, including auditory and somatosensory.

Auditory hallucinations can be of single voices or choirs; there is often a religious component. The voices are not persecutory and do not give a commentary on the patient. They are thus distinct from those found in schizophrenia.

Somatosensory hallucinations can be of people brushing past or of a touch on the skin. Patients and carers do not always describe all the forms of hallucination experienced; somatosensory hallucinations are rarely declared voluntarily.

The degree of insight into the hallucinations is variable. Many patients believe in the hallucination at the time but realize later that it could not be true. Some patients remain certain that the hallucinations are real and some realize they are unreal even as they look at them.

13.10 Can DLB present with purely visual problems?

A few patients with DLB present with problems exclusively with higher visual function. They complain of difficulties with their vision, which they find hard to characterize. They have difficulty locating objects on a table and finding their way around. With patience, they usually perform well on tests of visual acuity and therefore often puzzle opticians and ophthalmologists. On testing, they will fail to pick out the correct coin from a series and have difficulty locating their hands when testing visual fields. More formal testing of visual processing, such as clock-drawing or identifying incomplete letters, show marked deficits. This variant is called posterior cortical atrophy. It is a selective atrophy that can often be seen on an MRI scan (*Fig. 13.1*).

There are only two common causes of posterior cortical atrophy – DLB and Alzheimer's disease.

13.11 What is the relationship between DLB and Alzheimer's disease?

This is not a straightforward question and there is considerable disagreement between experts.

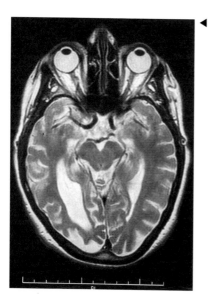

Fig. 13.1 Focal atrophy of the occipital and parietal lobes on an MRI scan is more marked on the right in a patient with clinical Alzheimer's disease presenting with visual disorientation.

Some patients with clinical DLB definitely do not have Alzheimer's disease. These patients have prominent hallucinations, fluctuations, parkinsonism and myoclonus. Other patients who present with memory and visuospatial problems, and mild executive disorders, could have either Alzheimer's disease or DLB. The two diseases are distinct at opposite ends of the spectrum but some cases show intermediate features.

A similar argument applies to the pathological diagnosis: many patients with DLB show numerous Lewy bodies and might have senile plaques but lack the associated tau staining seen in Alzheimer's disease. If there are tangles they tend to have a different distribution to Alzheimer's disease, for example sparing the hippocampus. However, some intermediate patients show features of both diseases, with Lewy bodies, neurofibrillary tangles and amyloid plaques.

The arguments between experts will be resolved when more is known of the pathogenesis of DLB and Alzheimer's disease.

13.12 Are there clinical features that can distinguish those patients with a parkinsonian syndrome who will later develop DLB?

The parkinsonian features of DLB are very similar to those of Parkinson's disease. There are a number of differences from idiopathic Parkinson's disease:

- patients suffer with drug-induced visual hallucinations at an early stage
- tremor is less prominent
- patients respond less well and in a less sustained way to dopaminergic agents
- patients often suffer with sudden jerks – myoclonus.

None of these differences is a certain discriminator between the two related conditions.

13.13 If a patient has both a dementia and parkinsonism is this always DLB?

No, there are a very large number of other diseases in which dementia and parkinsonism occur together, including cerebrovascular disease and other neurodegenerative diseases (e.g. corticobasal degeneration, progressive supranuclear palsy and Alzheimer's disease). Neuroleptic medication in virtually any late-onset neurodegenerative disease is prone to give parkinsonian side-effects. There are also numerous genetic diseases in which parkinsonism and dementia are seen together, including Wilson's disease, early-onset Huntington's disease (the Westphal variant) (see Q 13.24) and Hallervorden–Spatz disease. Some of these genetic causes are discussed in more detail in Chapter 14.

13.14 What is a typical case history for DLB?

CASE STUDY

Henry Fakenham is a 64-year-old banker. He took early retirement 2 years ago and at the time there was a feeling that he was no longer as good at taking decisions and managing the business. Since retirement he has been apathetic and has not pursued his hobbies of gardening and walking as his wife thought he would. He also began to see his GP regularly complaining of headaches for which no cause was found.

While staying in a hotel in France he saw an angel-like figure by his bedside, which he described to his wife; at the time he felt the figure was real but he now recognizes it as a hallucination. At times he appears disorientated and at other times his old self. He has continued to hallucinate, sometimes seeing the same angel and sometimes less well-defined figures around his bed. He has complained about other people being in the house and at times feels people brush past him when no-one is there.

His handwriting, which used to be large and clear, has become small but neat. He is less dextrous than he used to be at doing up buttons and he has slowed in his walk and stoops a little. His GP referred him to a neurologist when he found him disorientated, suspecting a brain tumour, but when seen the following week Henry was much improved and there was little to find on physical examination apart from mild parkinsonism. An MRI scan was reported as mild generalized atrophy.

13.15 What do investigations show in DLB/PD?

The diagnosis of DLB/PD remains a clinical one. Laboratory and other investigations in these patients are aimed at excluding other causes for the symptoms, rather than confirming the diagnosis.

Neuroimaging using either CT or MRI can either be normal or can show atrophy. The atrophy might be generalized or selectively involve the parietal and frontal lobes. Patients with a posterior cortical syndrome with marked visual problems often have occipital lobe atrophy visible on their scans (*Fig. 13.1*). Sparing of the hippocampi in a patient with advanced dementia is more in keeping with DLB/PD than Alzheimer's disease.

Cerebrospinal fluid protein, glucose and cell counts are normal. The EEG usually shows generally mild generalized slowing.

13.16 What treatments are available for DLB/PD?

The non-drug treatments for DLB/PD are discussed in Chapter 5. Drug therapy is either generally aimed at improving the cognitive symptoms or aimed at improving the parkinsonian symptoms. Unfortunately many drugs that improve the parkinsonian features of DLB/PD can worsen the cognitive problems, and vice versa. The introduction of l-dopa or dopamine agonists can produce increased behavioural problems. The use of neuroleptics (including the newer, atypical ones) for behavioural problems in DLB can lead to severe (sometimes life-threatening) worsening of the parkinsonian features.

There are no licensed drugs at present for the memory problems seen in DLB/PD but the cholinesterase inhibitors rivastigmine, donezepil and galantamine seem to more effective in DLB than in Alzheimer's disease. They can fulfill a very useful role in DLB, often improving the attention and behaviour of patients. Although, theoretically, cholinesterase inhibitors might be expected to worsen the motor features of DLB/PD, this is not usually a clinical problem. However, there is a problem with prescribing cholinesterase inhibitors in the UK at present because they are not licensed for use in DLB. This should change in the future with the increasing evidence in their favour, but at present their prescription should be initiated by a specialist.

Behavioural problems sometimes need specific treatment and the neuroleptics are discussed in Chapter 6.

13.17 How should I treat the motor problems of DLB?

Treating the parkinsonian features of DLB with dopaminergic agents can lead to increased visual hallucinations, disorientation and agitation. Nevertheless, once patients are significantly disabled with their parkinsonian features they generally benefit from dopaminergic agents.

There is no good-quality evidence to prove that the older dopa preparations (e.g. Sinemet and Madopar) are better than the newer dopamine agonists but generally the older drugs are more effective and have fewer side-effects. It is important to start at low doses – even as low as 50 mg dopa per day and build up over a month to a reasonable dose of 300 mg a day. Many patients do better on a combination of dopa and a cholinesterase inhibitor or neuroleptic than on no medication. Indeed, patients with severe parkinsonian problems need L-dopa to function. The newer dopa agonists can be tried but try to avoid combination therapy (L-dopa plus dopamine agonist) in patients who have severe cognitive problems. There are several other therapeutic options: all can worsen confusion – should generally be prescribed by a specialist.

■ Selegilene was once prescribed for virtually every patient with Parkinson's disease on the basis that it improved the prognosis of the disease. It was then prescribed for virtually none after evidence of a possible excess mortality when the drug was combined with L-dopa. It has now made a modest comeback and gives mild antiparkinsonian action with few side-effects.

■ Amantidine also has a mild antiparkinsonian effect and is a mild antidepressant. It is therefore sometimes useful but it can worsen hallucinations.

■ Anticholinergics such as benzhexol can help the tremor of Parkinson's disease but might also worsen confusion. They should generally be avoided in patients with significant cognitive problems and used with caution in patients at risk of becoming confused (e.g. the elderly).

13.18 How should I modify the treatment of patients with Parkinson's disease with dementia?

The approach needed to treat the motor problems of Parkinson's disease with dementia is different to that used to treat patients presenting with DLB because Parkinson's disease patients are nearly always on dopaminergic therapy prior to the development of cognitive problems. Nowadays, patients tend to be on combination therapy with an L-dopa preparation and a dopamine agonist.

 Dopamine agonists probably cause more confusion for less benefit than L-dopa and can be gradually withdrawn/replaced with l-dopa. It is important to avoid a sudden withdrawal of the drugs because this often results in the patient becoming rigid and immobile. If the patient and partner are managing there might be no need to change but when hallucinations or behavioural problems need to be tackled it is worth trying to:

- Reduce the amount of dopa the patient has in the late afternoon or evening because hallucinations tend to occur in the evening.
- Simplify the regime. Try to keep the patient on one sort of l-dopa preparation rather than several. Many patients are on regimes that mix two or more types of l-dopa preparation and have become very complex with the many changes that have accumulated over the years. On these regimes it becomes impossible to guess what the drug levels are at any point in the day. The simplest method is to change to an ordinary Sinemet or Madopar (125 mg) every 2–4 hours as necessary. If the patient is well established on slow release, or prefers slow release, this can be given every 3–6 hours. If the patient has swallowing problems then dispersible Madopar preparations are useful.
- Add a cholinesterase inhibitor, which often improves the behavioural problems, disorientation and hallucinations with little effect on the mobility. The dose needs to be titrated up slowly. This treatment should be supervised by a specialist.

Drugs are sometimes indicated for other problems associated with DLB/PD. Myoclonus can be a very troublesome feature of DLB and several drugs can help, including valproate (starting at 200 mg tds) or clonazepam (starting at a dose of 0.5 mg daily); clonazepam is often poorly tolerated in patients with dementia but some patients do well with it.

13.19 If a neuroleptic has to be used in DLB/PD, which is the best?

 The parkinsonian side-effects of neuroleptics are well known and most patients on a high dose of neuroleptics will develop some parkinsonian side-effects. However, patients with DLB/PD are much more sensitive to the side-effects and any introduction of a neuroleptic must be evaluated carefully. Some patients with DLB become very stiff and rigid on small doses of prochlorperazine and, if not recognized, this can lead to severe disability. It is not unusual for patients with DLB/PD to need hospitalization as a result of the introduction of a neuroleptic. Another reason to be cautious is that it is not unusual for patients with DLB/PD to take months to recover from a regular neuroleptic regime. However, despite these caveats, neuroleptics are sometimes needed in DLB/PD.

It is worth a specialist considering a cholinesterase inhibitor prior to neuroleptic treatment. Some patients with DLB are so behaviourally disturbed that without a neuroleptic they would need long-term care. The conventional neuroleptics such as chlorpromazine and haloperidol can cause severe parkinsonian side-effects. When the atypical antipsychotics olanzapine and respiridone were first introduced it was felt that they had minimal extrapyramidal side-effects and they became the drugs of choice in DLB/PD. Unfortunately, many patients with DLB do have marked worsening of their parkinsonian features with these drugs. Clozapine still has a place but it needs careful haematological monitoring. One of the newest drugs quetiapine is thought to be relatively free of extrapyramidal effects and is being used increasingly. Otherwise, olanzapine is probably the best choice, although many psychiatrists prefer respiridone.

There is still a role for the older drugs: neurologists often choose sulpiride because it seems to cause less worsening of parkinsonian features than most.

13.20 What abnormalities are seen in the MMSE and ACE in DLB/PD?

The typical problems seen on the MMSE are similar to those seen in Alzheimer's disease, although tests of attention such as the serial 7s might be affected rather earlier.

On the ACE, the earliest problems tend to be with verbal fluency or visuospatial tasks. Some patients with DLB have early problems with anterograde memory (recall of the learnt address) similar to those seen in Alzheimer's disease, but more typically they have more difficulty registering the address than recalling it. Overall, it would be a bold clinician who tried confidently to distinguish Alzheimer's disease and DLB/PD on the MMSE or the ACE, unless the small handwriting (micrographia) in the written sentence gives the diagnosis away.

13.21 What does neuropsychological testing show in DLB?

The first abnormalities seen in patients with DLB on neuropsychological testing are problems with attention and concentration. These can be tested for by the Trails test, which is a sophisticated version of a child's dot-to-dot puzzle.

There is also early evidence of problems with tests of executive function and problem solving on the Wisconsin Card Sorting test and the Tower of London test (*see Q 12.17* for a description of these tests).

Some patients with DLB have similar problems with anterograde and episodic memory as those seen in Alzheimer's disease and will do poorly on recall of the Rey figure (*see Q 2.31*) and with delayed recall of a passage.

Visuospatial skills are usually impaired and this can be the presenting or the dominant feature; the patient might have great difficulty even copying the Rey figure and recognizing simple line drawings.

13.22 What psychiatric problems occur with DLB/PD?

Psychiatric problems are more common in DLB than in Alzheimer's disease and in a small minority of cases they can be the presenting feature. The diagnosis of DLB in such patients is difficult in the early stages of the disease. A clue emerges when patients become very parkinsonian when treated with neuroleptic drugs. The psychiatric presentations of DLB can take several forms:

- Hypochondriasis: late-onset hypochondriasis can be a presenting feature of DLB. Patients might complain vociferously about certain problems and cannot be persuaded that there is no serious underlying cause (and in this case they are right). Patients sometimes claim they cannot walk when clearly they can.
- Other delusional beliefs, which can be persistent.
- Depression: severe depression and suicide can occur in the early stages of DLB. It can be accompanied by anxiety.
- Hallucinations: the hallucinations of DLB can be mistaken for late-onset psychoses. The auditory hallucinations are the most likely to lead to a psychiatric referral. The hallucinations of DLB are usually not threatening and can be pleasant.
- Disorientation and agitation: can lead to a psychiatric referral.

These problems, together with aggression and wandering, can cause considerable problems later in the disease and are a particular problem in patients taking dopaminergic drugs for their parkinsonian symptoms.

13.23 What is the course and prognosis of DLB?

The prognosis of DLB is rather variable. Some patients present with a rapidly progressive dementia with florid psychiatric problems and dramatic fluctuations in cognition and orientation. Such patients are often referred early to neurologists with a suspicion of tumours or prion disease (see

Chapter 16). Unlike prion disease, after the initial rapid deterioration, patients with DLB often plateau for a period before deteriorating slowly in a similar fashion to other degenerative dementias. Patients who develop mild cognitive problems after having Parkinson's disease often have a relatively benign course. Overall, the prognosis is similar to Alzheimer's disease with the average patient living for about 7 years after diagnosis.

HUNTINGTON'S DISEASE

13.24 What is Huntington's disease?

Huntington's disease is the most common genetic cause of dementia. Many individuals know that they are at risk of developing the disease and therefore the diagnosis is usually straightforward. However, a surprising number present with no family history and Huntington's disease therefore needs to be considered in patients with an unusual dementia, particularly with an early age of onset or a movement disorder.

Huntington's disease is an autosomal dominant disease that can present from any age from childhood to old age. In childhood it often starts with an atypical parkinsonian syndrome – the so-called Westphal variant.

In adults, Huntington's disease can present with a movement disorder or with cognitive problems. The movement disorder is chorea, which is characterized by quick, unpredictable, jerky movements. Patients seek to disguise the chorea by making the choreic jerk into an action, for example brushing their hair. In the early stages of the disease, patients appear very restless and fidgety. Later, the larger, virtually continuous movements become obvious. Patients might not complain of the movement and relatives might not notice anything new.

The cognitive problems are predominantly subcortical, with slowing of thought becoming apparent with time. Although, given long enough, patients will often give the correct answer to a question. There is also a personality change, with increased apathy. Depression is very common in Huntington's disease and can be the presenting feature. It often complicates the assessment of the patient's memory.

13.25 What physical signs are seen in Huntington's disease?

Physical examination nearly always reveals abnormalities in Huntington's disease in the early stages. The chorea is often first seen as fidgetiness. It can be made more obvious by distracting patients – it is often visible in the hands when the patient walks. When patients are given a mental task that requires concentration, such as reciting the months of the year backwards, the chorea becomes more apparent. Patients are unable to keep their tongue protruded for 10 seconds without withdrawing it. The eye movements are usually abnormal, although this can be very subtle. Usually, the first sign is slowing of the fast voluntary vertical eye movements (the saccades). Vertical saccades can be examined by the physician holding one hand midway between the patient and the examiner's chest and the other above the patient's head, and asking the patient to look quickly from one hand to the other.

Other features can include parkinsonian features, poor balance and dysarthria.

13.26 What is a typical history for Huntington's disease?

CASE STUDY

Rachel Gayton is 34 years old. She feels that she has few problems but her husband feels that she no longer looks after the children with the care that she used to. She has been depressed for the last 2 years and this has not responded to treatment with an antidepressant. Friends and family also complain that she fidgets non-stop. Her father left her mother when he was 38 years old and nothing further was heard from him, but there is no other family history.

On examination, as she walks Rachel makes little quick grimaces and hand flicks; she is also unable to sit still. She is rather withdrawn and slow. Vertical eye saccades are broken and she cannot hold her tongue protruded for more than a couple of seconds.

The possibility of Huntington's disease is mentioned to the family and at her next consultation Rachel's mother also comes. It becomes clear that she had heard that her husband was admitted to a psychiatric ward after the divorce and that his mother had also died in a mental hospital with a possible diagnosis of Huntington's disease. Genetic testing shows that Rachel does have the typical triplet repeat expansion of Huntington's disease.

13.27 How is Huntington's disease diagnosed?

The diagnosis of Huntington's disease is usually made in one of two scenarios. The first is in individuals who know that they are at risk of developing the disease and begin to develop symptoms. If the examination reveals chorea or evidence of cognitive problems then the diagnosis becomes very likely. The second scenario is patients presenting without a family history of Huntington's disease. The presentation is usually with chorea, depression or cognitive changes.

The crucial test is to look for evidence of the mutation that causes Huntington's disease in the patient's blood. An ordinary blood sample can be used and the mutation screened by a genetic laboratory. The presence of the mutation establishes that the individual is at risk of developing Huntington's disease and, if they have relevant symptoms and signs, establishes the diagnosis.

13.28 What is the Huntington's mutation?

The mutation lies on the short arm of chromosome 4 and is in a gene that codes for the protein huntingtin. The normal huntingtin gene has a sequence of base pairs in which has the sequence cytosine, adenosine and guanine are repeated up to 30 times – a so-called CAG repeat. The number of CAG repeats any individual has on each of their two chromosomes varies. If the number of repeats increases over the generations until there are more than 35–40 then the patient has a very high chance of developing Huntington's disease and the disease will be passed on in that individual's genes. The more repeats there are, the more likely an individual is to develop the disease earlier in life. Because the triple sequence is repeated in the mutation, the mutation is often described as a triplet repeat or triplet expansion mutation.

13.29 How is the gene passed on?

The Huntington's mutation is passed on in an autosomal dominant fashion, which means that the child of an individual carrying the mutation has a 50% chance of receiving the mutation. The disease gene shows high penetrance – if you have the mutation then it is very likely that you will develop the disease if you live long enough.

There is a tendency for the mutation to expand in size if it is passed on from father to child. Thus individuals who inherit the gene from their father tend to develop the disease at an earlier age than their father, this phenomenon is called anticipation; it is characteristic of triplet repeat mutation diseases. The triplet repeat mutation does not usually expand if the disease is passed on by the mother.

13.30 How accurate is genetic testing?

Genetic testing for Huntington's disease is very sensitive and specific. There were some problems in the early days but these are now extremely rare. Patients who have a dementia or chorea and who carry the mutation will virtually always have Huntington's disease. If two alleles have been amplified in the genetics laboratory and neither have the expansion mutation then the patient does not have Huntington's disease.

When the disease gene was first located, all the families with suspected Huntington's disease were tested and virtually all were positive. However, there are occasional families with a Huntington's-like phenotype who do not carry the disease gene, but these are very few and, when examined, are usually atypical.

13.31 Does a patient who carries the mutation need further investigation such as scanning?

As a general rule, patients do not require the tests they would have for other forms of dementia. However, the possibility of dual pathology needs to be considered and, for example, a patient with Huntington's disease who was deteriorating rapidly after a head injury might require a CT scan to exclude the possibility of an additional subdural haematoma.

13.32 Why is there no family history of Huntington's disease in some individuals?

Initially, it is surprising how often Huntington's disease is diagnosed in individuals who have no family history of the disease. There are a number of possible reasons for this:

- the family history was known to the previous generation but, because of the shame attached to the diagnosis, it was never discussed
- the disease was misdiagnosed in the parents. The most common misdiagnoses include brain tumours, dementia and Parkinson's disease
- the individual in the previous generation died of some other cause before showing signs of the disease
- the family has split up and nothing is known (usually of the father). This is more common in families in which Huntington's disease is inherited – due to the personality and other changes early in the disease
- the disease is the result of a new mutation (this is very rare) or because of anticipation the disease had only very mild or no effects in the father
- non-paternity.

13.33 Do I need to refer patients for genetic counselling prior to testing for the Huntington's mutation?

In many ways, the genetic test is little different from hundreds of other diagnostic tests that doctors perform. However, the Huntington's test is more precise than many and does have consequences for other family members. It is therefore important to talk to the patient and to relatives prior to performing the genetic test for Huntington's disease. If the patient has symptoms then it is usually more appropriate for a doctor with knowledge of Huntington's disease to counsel the patient and the family. They need to be told the consequences of a positive diagnosis. If there are clear family disagreements or other problems over whether an affected individual should be tested then it is usually wise to involve a medical genetics specialist before doing the genetic test.

Relatives of affected individual who are asymptomatic and wish to be tested to see if they carry the disease gene are a very different prospect and should be referred to a specialist in medical genetics before genetic testing.

13.34 Which patients in Huntington's families should I refer to a neurologist and which to a geneticist?

> Families who know they are affected often have a close relationship with a geneticist or neurologist and so this question does not arise. If it does, then as a rule of thumb those who are showing symptoms and signs should be referred to a neurologist and those without symptoms who want advice or testing should be referred to a geneticist.

13.35 I have a patient at risk of developing Huntington's disease who wishes to be tested for the disease. What should I advise?

Individuals at risk of developing Huntington's disease who are considering being tested should see a consultant in medical genetics.

There are arguments for and against testing for the disease gene. There is a risk of depression and other psychological reactions to the test result whether it is positive or negative. A negative result should never be given lightly. Some patients have lived for many years with the knowledge that they have a high chance of developing a fatal disease and have lived their life accordingly. The sudden removal of this, and the realization that they have to plan for a full and normal life, can have unexpected consequences.

Patients who want to know if they carry the disease gene for a clear reason (e.g. deciding whether to have children) will often have testing. The point of testing someone just to predict the future is less clear.

13.36 How does Huntington's disease progress?

Huntington's disease is slowly progressive and the patient gradually becomes increasingly dysarthric and might eventually become mute. Swallowing problems are often prominent and might necessitate insertion of a percutaneous gastrostomy tube. Balance and gait deteriorate and patients usually need increasing help to walk and will often become confined to a wheelchair. The physical problems often make assessment of the dementia difficult. The cognitive changes also progress and patients become increasingly apathetic and amnesic.

Depression is often a prominent feature and can be resistant to treatment.

13.37 Is treatment available for Huntington's disease?

The chorea is treatable. The drug of first choice is often tetrabenazine. Unfortunately, this has a number of side-effects, including drowsiness and depression, and these often limits its use. A number of other drugs can improve the chorea, including anticholinergics such as benzhexol and neuroleptics such as sulpiride, but these also have significant side-effects. Patients are often not too troubled with the chorea and prefer to leave it untreated rather than suffer the side-effects of the medication.

The cognitive problems are not usually treatable and no trials of cholinesterase inhibitors have been reported in Huntington's disease. However, donepezil and rivastigmine often improve attention and might be effective.

13.38 Are there any forms of treatment for Huntington's under development?

Huntington's disease is a common genetic disease that is always progressive and eventually fatal. It is therefore imperative to try to develop more effective treatments to prevent the disease or alter its course. A number of more invasive treatments are under development. One of the aims of molecular biology is to establish a new way of treating genetic diseases through genetic cures. These treatments aim to repair the defective gene that causes a disease or replace the defective gene with a normal one. Huntington's disease as one of the more common fatal genetic diseases is a focus of research attention. However, there are still problems in finding a way of incorporating normal genes into the cells in the caudate and elsewhere in the brain.

Trials of transplants of tissue into the brains of affected individuals are also under way. Suitable cells are taken from the adrenal glands of fetuses aborted for medical reasons and then prepared and transplanted into the caudates of patients with Huntington's disease. Early work suggests that such techniques are safe and result in survival of the graft but it is too early to know whether they will be an effective treatment.

13.39 Do any other diseases cause a combination of chorea and dementia?

Yes. The more common ones include:

- cerebral lupus, particularly associated with the lupus anticoagulant and anticardiolipin antibodies
- variant Creutzfeldt–Jakob disease
- cerebrovascular disease
- other genetic diseases such as dentatorubralpallidolysial atrophy (DRPLA).

Hyperthyroidism can also cause a combination of chorea and cognitive changes.

PATIENT QUESTIONS

13.40 Do all patients who hallucinate on L-dopa preparations have DLB?

No. Hallucinations are a common side-effect of L-dopa preparations; more common still are vivid dreams. Hallucinations alone should not lead to a diagnosis of DLB/PD, especially if they go when the medication is changed or stopped. It is when hallucinations occur with other cognitive symptoms that a dementia becomes likely. Some patients have hallucinations that settle or stay stable for many years without any cognitive problems. It is not known whether patients who have hallucinations early in the disease process are more likely to develop DLB later.

13.41 Who develops DLB?

DLB is mainly a disease of people over the age of 50 years, although younger people develop it occasionally. It is more common in men than women. There are a few reported familial cases but in the vast majority of cases it is sporadic.

13.42 My husband has DLB. Will he have passed it to our children or grandchildren?

Compared with other forms of degenerative dementia, relatively few patients with DLB have a family history of dementia. A few familial cases have been reported but are rare compared with Alzheimer's disease and FTD. The vast majority of cases of DLB are therefore sporadic and you can be reassured that your children and grandchildren are very unlikely to develop the disease.

13.43 Is DLB the same as the Lewy body variant of Alzheimer's disease, diffuse Lewy body disease or cortical Lewy body disease?

These names all refer to the same disease, an international agreement has settled on the name 'dementia with Lewy bodies' for patients whose dementia starts before or within a year of the onset of Parkinson's disease and Parkinson's disease with dementia for patients with a longer history of Parkinson's disease prior to developing dementia.

13.44 How does DLB start?

DLB can start in a number of different ways:

- with difficulties planning tasks, generally 'slowing down' and forgetting very recent events
- with a combination of hallucinations – seeing people, animals or objects that are not there. These might be combined with difficulty finding routes or looking for an object on a table and just not seeing it
- with predominantly psychiatric problems – depression, abnormal thoughts or hypochondiasis.

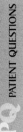

These problems can occur before any signs of Parkinson's disease or can develop in a patient diagnosed as having Parkinson's disease.

13.45 What causes DLB?

This remains unknown. Indeed, the causes of the majority of cases of Parkinson's disease are unclear. Inherited cases are very unusual and therefore it seems likely that environmental factors play a major role. The actual environmental triggers remain to be found.

13.46 I am 50 years old, my aunt (father's sister) developed Huntington's disease at the age of 54. What are my chances of developing the disease?

A number of factors determine the risk. You share 1 in 4 of your aunt's genes but your actual risk is less than this for a number of reasons. The most important factor for you is your father's health. If your father is still alive and well then he probably does not carry the disease gene and you are likely to be fine. However, if your father died young, your risk is higher. Also if you are now 50 years old then you are partially through the age of risk and your risk is less than 1 in 4.

For a personal risk assessment you need to see a medical geneticist.

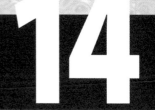

Dementia and other neurological diseases

MULTIPLE SCLEROSIS (MS)

14.1 Can MS present with dementia?

Multiple sclerosis (MS) usually starts as a relapsing, remitting disease with an emphasis on eye, cerebellar and spinal cord symptoms. After a variable period, a proportion of patients develop progressive neurological problems. Cognitive problems are rare in the early stages of the disease, although if tested thoroughly minor abnormalities can be picked up on psychometric testing in a few patients.

There are a few patients with MS whose illness starts with cognitive problems; a larger number had undiagnosed or long-forgotten episodes of demyelination in the past who present anew with cognitive problems. The presentation is variable and the features can include:

- a progressive amnesia mimicking a degenerative dementia but often with features (e.g. urinary urgency and gait ataxia) that suggest a multisystem neurological problem
- cognitive problems accompanied by psychiatric features such as paranoia, mania, hallucinations or depression
- a frontal lobe syndrome with disinhibition or apathy.

Cognitive problems become more common in the progressive phase of MS. The typical problems are apathy and some slowing of cognition, sometimes combined with a mild inappropriate euphoria. As the physical problems from MS become greater so do the cognitive problems, and some patients develop a severe dementia. Dementia is common in patients with severe cerebellar disease and in those with pendular nystagmus.

The cognitive problems in MS usually occur very gradually and are usually slowly progressive. There are often clues to the diagnosis in the examination of the patient, including:

- gaze-evoked nystagmus or broken ocular pursuit movements
- internuclear ophthalmoplegia
- absent vibration sense in the feet
- mild limb or gait ataxia.

These abnormalities can occur in the absence of a history of motor or sensory problems.

14.2 What investigations are needed in suspected MS?

The usual investigations needed are an MRI scan of the brain and sometimes of the spinal cord. Patients with MS who have dementia usually have significant cerebral atrophy and periventricular white matter changes on their MRI brain scan. Lumbar puncture is usually needed in unusual presentations of MS, such as dementia, to examine the CSF for intrathecal synthesis of oligoclonal bands. If these are present only in the CSF (and not in the serum) the diagnosis of MS is more secure. Delay in the visual-evoked responses also supports the diagnosis of MS. A vitamin B_{12} estimation and autoantibody screen are important to exclude vitamin B_{12} deficiency or lupus.

The differential diagnosis of MS presenting with cognitive problems is wide and includes systemic lupus erythematosus (and the lupus anticoagulant syndrome), sarcoidosis, vasculitis, adrenoleucodystrophy and vitamin B_{12} deficiency.

14.3 Can the cognitive problems associated with MS be treated?

There is no specific treatment for the cognitive problems associated with MS. The newer agents, such as beta-interferon, CAMPATH (an antibody-mediated treatment for MS) and copolymer 1, have not been shown to be effective for the cognitive symptoms of MS. These symptoms are usually a feature of the progressive phase of the disease and the major therapeutic effect of the newer drugs is to reduce the number of relapses a patient suffers.

A major priority in treating patients with MS and memory problems is to consider depression. MS and depression often coexist and many patients with MS have complaints such as fatigue, poor concentration and amnesia, which could be caused by depression. The choice of antidepressant should be made on the same basis as in other patients. Amitriptyline (starting at a dose of 10 mg *nocte* and aiming for a dose of 50–75 mg daily) is a good choice for patients with somatic and cognitive symptoms, particularly if they are sleeping poorly. Patients who are apathetic or intolerant of side-effects might be better treated with an SSRI.

PROGRESSIVE SUPRANUCLEAR PALSY (PSP)

14.4 What is PSP?

Progressive supranuclear palsy (PSP) is a degenerative disease of the midbrain and cerebrum that was first described in the 1970s by a group of American neurologists and pathologists. Steele, Richardson and Olzwelski identified a group of patients with common clinical and pathological features. Their description led to the recognition of similar cases by neurologists throughout the world and many more patients were reported. The disease was originally called Steele–Richardson syndrome but PSP has become the accepted name.

The physical features of PSP are of a slowly progressive combination of visual difficulties (which often puzzle opticians), unsteadiness of gait, clumsiness of the limbs and difficulties with swallowing. These are often combined with a type of dementia in which patients become slow in their thoughts but 'get there in the end'.

14.5 Does PSP run in families?

Although it was initially felt that PSP was a purely sporadic disease, occasional families have been described who have PSP inherited as an autosomal dominant trait. However, the vast majority of cases are sporadic and families can usually be reassured that siblings and children are unlikely to develop similar problems. Occasional cases have been shown to be due to mutations in the tau gene (*see Q 12.24*); a certain form of the tau gene (called the Ao genotype) is common in patients with PSP. It is possible to type individuals and see if they are Ao positive but the Ao genotype is too common in the general population for this to be of use in the diagnosis of PSP.

14.6 What is the prognosis of PSP?

PSP is a more rapidly progressive disease than Parkinson's disease and patients usually become severely disabled within 2 years of onset. Early falls are characteristic and difficulties with walking and balance can lead to early confinement to a wheelchair. Difficulty with eating and speech are usually severe and often lead to the need for a 'lite writer' to aid communication and the insertion of a percutaneous feeding tube to maintain calorie intake. The eyeballs can become virtually static in their sockets. The physical handicaps often make assessment of cognitive function difficult and can lead to the underestimation or overestimation of the cognitive problems by carers and doctors.

14.7 What are the physical signs to look for in PSP?

On examination, patients have restricted eye movements, particularly when moving the eyes up and down, and the eyelids often retract to give a startled, staring expression. Patients have a dysarthria and a stiff neck, which is often held extended and twisted to one side (retrocollis and torticollis). The limbs are rigid as in Parkinson's disease and movements are slowed. Walking gait is often upright and unsteady.

The ocular palsy is called a supranuclear gaze palsy because the pathways that are damaged in the disease process come from the cerebrum and end at the oculomotor nerve nuclei (i.e. above the ocular nerve nuclei). Patients become unable to move the eyes to command, although they can make reflex or involuntary movements because the path from the oculomotor nerve nuclei to the ocular muscles is intact. This can be demonstrated clinically by asking patients to fix their eyes on an object. The examiner then moves the patient's head from side to side and up and down as the patient fixates the object. The eyes move in their sockets to remain fixed on the object. The neurological way of describing this is to say that 'doll's eye' movements are present. If this test is done with a patient in whom there is disease of the oculomotor nerves, then the eyes move passively with the head.

14.8 How is PSP diagnosed?

There is no specific test for PSP and the diagnosis is made on the basis of the history and examination. CT or MRI brain scans might show some atrophy of structures in the posterior fossa or the cerebral hemispheres but these findings are not specific. Many cases probably remain undiagnosed or misdiagnosed as atypical Parkinson's disease or cerebrovascular disease.

A number of atypical cases has been described. It is important to perform a brain scan in patients with PSP because occasional patients with a midbrain tumour or obstructive hydrocephalus can have similar clinical features.

14.9 What cognitive problems are seen in PSP?

Although PSP is sometimes regarded as a motor problem – a 'movement disorder' – the cognitive problems were recognized in early descriptions of the disease and can be the presenting feature of PSP. During the 1990s there was increasing interest in the cognitive problems of PSP and it is now recognized that PSP patients will sometimes present to a neurologist with cognitive problems and minimal motor complaints and signs. The typical feature of the dementia associated with PSP is a slowing of thought. Study of patients with PSP led to the concept of a subcortical dementia, in which the cerebral cortex works normally but the white matter connections between cortical cells do not. The slowing-down of messages between the different parts of the cortex results in a slowing of the thought process with few specific focal problems such as aphasia, etc.

In practice, it is very difficult to distinguish a subcortical dementia from some forms of frontal lobe dementia. Indeed, both frontal lobe disease and subcortical disease probably play a role in the dementia seen in PSP. Some patients with PSP do have a more cortical form of dementia with amnesia. A number of more specific deficits are now recognized in PSP, such as a naming difficulty for nouns.

14.10 Can PSP be treated?

Treatment of the parkinsonian features of PSP with L-dopa or other parkinsonian drugs is worthwhile. A number of patients do respond. However, the response is less good and less sustained than in Parkinson's disease. A reasonable regime would be to gradually introduce Madopar or Sinemet, aiming for a dose of 100–125 mg four times a day over a 4-week period. If there is no response and the drug is well tolerated, this dose can be doubled. If the L-dopa cannot be tolerated or has no effect, it should be withdrawn over a couple of weeks.

The dystonia of the neck or limbs is often responsive to botulinum toxin injections. These injections improve dystonia by selectively weakening those muscles that are overactive and which produce the twisting movement. The response to botulinum toxin usually lasts for 2–3 months. Repeated injections are therefore needed – the toxin usually retains its potency. Occasionally patients develop antibodies to the botulinum toxin but this can usually be treated by changing the preparation of toxin.

A number of patients with PSP respond to amantidine, a drug often used in Parkinson's disease. There is no convincing evidence of its efficacy and it is not licensed for PSP. However, it is often worth trying amantidine in PSP – a disease with a rapidly progressive course and little other treatment.

CORTICOBASAL DEGENERATION (CBD)

14.11 What is CBD?

Corticobasal degeneration (CBD) was first described in the mid-1980s. It usually starts insidiously when a patient develops problems with one limb, usually a hand. The hand will no longer perform skilled actions that used to be done automatically. A typical problem would be difficulty throwing up a tennis ball before serving. The action might be first noted when the patient is performing a particularly skilled task, such as a surgeon tying knots or a typist using a keyboard. The problems progress and all actions of the hand start to be affected. A characteristic feature is that the hand starts to do things by itself. It wanders away from the body and might start to interfere with the actions of the other hand. This is called the alien hand phenomenon. The problems gradually become worse and spread to the foot on the same side and then to the opposite arm. The foot drags when walking and will not perform complex actions. The affected limbs often give small irregular jerks – myoclonus. It becomes clear that the patient has a generalized neurodegenerative disease and features of Parkinson's disease and cerebellar disease develop. The initial descriptions minimized any cognitive problems but it is now apparent that, like PSP and motor neuron disease, in a minority of patients cognitive problems are significant, and in a subset of patients cognitive problems are the presenting feature.

14.12 What is the clinical presentation of CBD?

The clinical presentation of the cognitive problems is variable. The most typical problem is apraxia. Indeed, the presentation with an uncooperative limb is a sign of apraxia. A frontal syndrome is common, with personality change and difficulty planning complex tasks. Some patients develop an amnesia and visuospatial problems, and others present with a dementia, either with personality and behavioural change reminiscent of FTD or with more global cognitive problems.

Rare familial cases have been described, sometimes with a mutation in the tau gene, but CBD is generally a sporadic disease and in the absence of a family history, relatives of an affected individual should be reassured.

The treatment of CBD is difficult. Patients with parkinsonian features might respond to L-dopa in a similar fashion to patients with PSP, that is, less reliably and with a less sustained response than in Parkinson's disease.

14.13 What physical signs are found in CBD?

On examination, the patient might have a supranuclear gaze palsy similar to the one seen in PSP (*see Q 14.7*). There can be axial rigidity. The most striking problems are in the affected hand, which shows marked apraxia – difficulty in performing and copying postures, actions and gestures – despite the absence of gross weakness or other motor problems. The hand often jerks irregularly and can move off when the patient does not wish it to, particularly if the patient's attention is distracted. The limbs may be dystonic, with abnormal postures of the limb. The hand will not obey voluntary commands promptly and is clumsy. Basic sensory testing is often normal but more complex testing that requires a cortical input, such as two-point discrimination, are affected. On examination the patient will often have mild parkinsonian features, gait ataxia and pyramidal signs.

Examination of cognitive skills usually reveals a mild dysexecutive syndrome but some patients have more widespread cognitive problems.

LEUKODYSTROPHY

14.14 What is leukodystrophy?

'Leukodystrophy' means white matter disease. The white matter consists of the axons connecting the nerve cells and is concentrated in the cerebrum, where the axons connect different parts of the cortex and the two hemispheres of the brain. The term 'leukodystrophy' is used to describe a number of mainly genetic diseases in which the white matter is predominantly affected.

Many of the leukodystrophies are diagnosed in childhood when a child fails to develop normally and shows motor and cognitive delay. However, a number present in adulthood, occasionally when an individual presents to a memory clinic with cognitive problems. The typical cognitive syndrome is of slowing of thought processes and memory loss. The patient usually has other signs of white matter disease on examination – optic pallor secondary to demyelination of the optic nerves and pyramidal and posterior column signs (loss of vibration sense and joint position sense) in the legs. Some of the leukodystrophies are accompanied by a peripheral neuropathy.

14.15 What are the features of adrenoleukodystrophy?

One of the more common forms of leukodystrophy seen in adults is adrenoleukodystrophy, which also affects the adrenal glands. It is a sex-linked disease affecting men, although a milder form is seen in female 'carriers'. Usually a disease of childhood, it can present with a myelopathy and neuropathy in early adult life. These features are usually accompanied by a mild dementia. Very rarely, it presents in middle life with a dementia often with prominent visuospatial problems, these can include difficulty with route finding and identifying where objects are. Brain imaging and neurophysiology (such as visual evoked responses) often reveal evidence of white matter disease. The condition can be diagnosed by screening the blood for the ratio of very-long-chain fatty acids. This is the form of leukodystrophy for which Lorenzo's oil was suggested as a treatment, but its use in adults has been disappointing. Although a late-onset disease, adrenoleukodystrophy in adults can be rapidly progressive.

MITOCHONDRIAL DISEASE

14.16 What is mitochondrial disease?

Mitochondria are the organelles that provide the energy a cell needs to function. Mitochondria behave like microorganisms, living within a cell and dividing separately from the remainder of the cell. They are passed solely from the mother to the child; the paternal mitochondria in the sperm are either never admitted into the ova or quickly expelled. Some mitochondrial genes are encoded within the mitochondrion itself. Mutations within these genes tend to lead to inefficient respiration and dysfunction of the cells. Some cells are frequently affected by the mitochondrial dysfunction, others appear resistant. Neurons and muscle cells are often affected and typical features of mitochondrial disease include deafness, muscular weakness, cardiomyopathy, encephalopathy, renal failure and retinal disease. There are many associated features, including diabetes, short stature and lactic acidosis. The inheritance of most mitochondrial disease is maternal – it is passed to children by their mother but not by the father – reflecting the origin of the mitochondria.

Mitochondrial disease is one of the more common causes of dementia that develops in the teens and early adult life, although it can occur at any age. It is very rare for dementia to be the only feature and patients have other mitochondrial problems, such as deafness and diabetes. It is more common for patients to present with other features of mitochondrial disease, such as stroke-like episodes, a myopathy, diabetes or a cardiomyopathy, and for cognitive problems to emerge with time. There is no proven treatment for most forms of mitochondrial disease but men can usually be reassured that they are very unlikely to pass the disease onto their children.

EPILEPSY

14.17 Does epilepsy cause dementia?

There are a number of associations between epilepsy and dementia:

■ The two most common forms of dementia – Alzheimer's disease and vascular dementia – are associated with seizures, although seizures are common in Alzheimer's disease and are usually few in number. Several of the less common forms of dementia, including some of the treatable forms (e.g. brain tumours), are associated with seizures that can be more troublesome.

■ Seizures can result in temporary memory problems and many patients with epilepsy are aware that they have memory problems. Memory problems are most typically associated with temporal lobe epilepsy but occur in all forms.

■ Many of the major known causes of epilepsy, such as trauma, hippocampal disease and birth anoxia, are also associated with memory problems.

■ Long-term usage of some drugs such as the barbiturates can be associated with memory problems. Other drugs can cause cognitive problems as a toxic side-effect, especially at higher doses.

14.18 Which anticonvulsant should I use in a patient with dementia?

There is no good evidence favouring any of the anticonvulsants in dementia. Therefore the same anticonvulsants should be used as in other elderly individuals. Carbamazepine is the drug of choice provided there is adequate supervision to allow slow titration of the dose upwards. It is normal to start at a dose of 100 mg twice daily and gradually increase in 200 mg aliquots to 400 mg twice daily over 4 weeks. A slower rate of increase is fine if there are side-effects. Valproate has the advantage of quicker and easier titration and is a good alternative, starting at 300 mg bd and increasing to 500 mg bd after 2 weeks. Some patients with dementia cannot tolerate these normal doses and need smaller ones.

14.19 What is the typical memory problem in epilepsy?

The most typical memory problem seen in epilepsy is rapid forgetting, in which memories appear to be laid down normally and indeed events of the last few days can be recalled normally or nearly normally – the problem is with longer recall of events. Typical problems that arise with this form of amnesia are failure to recall major family events that took place a few months previously or an inability to recall the details of when and where holiday photographs were taken. Rapid forgetting is not screened for in psychometric testing and therefore psychometric results can be completely normal.

Many patients with rapid forgetting have frequent complex partial or generalized seizures and it was hoped that by vigorously treating the epilepsy the patient's memory could be improved. Although this happens in some patients, others seem to deteriorate or remain stable despite improved seizure control. Nevertheless, it is important to try to improve seizure control.

Some patients present with rapid forgetting without any clear clinical seizures and some of these show spikes on the EEG originating in the temporal lobes. A trial of an anticonvulsant such as carbamazepine is worthwhile in these patients.

CANCER

14.20 What are the causes of dementia in patients with cancer?

Cancer can produce dementia in three main ways:

- The cancer can affect the brain directly through primary or metastatic spread. The common tumours that spread to the brain include lung cancer, breast cancer and lymphoma.
- Metabolic problems caused by the cancer – thiamine deficiency or hypercalcaemia can cause cognitive problems.
- Antibodies produced by the body to fight the tumour can attack the nervous system and lead to dementia. The syndromes produced by these antibodies are called paraneoplastic syndromes.

14.21 Which paraneoplastic syndromes are associated with dementia?

There are several paraneoplastic syndromes but the two that cause dementia are progressive multifocal leukoencephalopathy (PML) and limbic encephalitis. Treatment of paraneoplastic syndromes is often disappointing, although patients might stop deteriorating – or even improve – if the primary tumour can be identified and treated. Immunoglobulins have been tried and there are some reports of success.

If a paraneoplastic syndrome is diagnosed then it is necessary to investigate for a primary tumour, including lung and gynaecological tumours and lymphoma.

14.22 What is progressive multifocal leukencephalopathy?

Progressive multifocal leukencephalopathy is a disease of the white matter associated with infection by the JC virus. It occurs in patients in Aids and other causes of immunodeficiency such as malignancy and drugs. It usually presents with a rapidly progressive dementia with problems with visual processing. The cognitive problems tend to progress over weeks. The patient becomes apathetic, forgetful and might develop limb problems, for example a hemiplegia or hemisensory loss. The diagnosis is usually made by MRI or CT scan, which will show confluent white-matter lesions affecting the subcortical and periventricular regions. Analysis of the CSF often shows a few lymphocytes with a mildly raised protein and sometimes oligoclonal bands. Although serological tests can be performed on the serum and CSF to try to confirm the diagnosis, these can be inconclusive. Brain biopsy is sometimes performed to try to make a diagnosis but can also be inconclusive.

The Aids-related variant of PML can be treated with HAART or other antiretroviral therapy. There are also reports of response to ganciclovir or cidofovir. PML associated with malignancy or other diseases has not been shown to be responsive to any treatment. The prognosis is poor and most patients die of the complications of dementia and immobility in 6–12 months.

14.23 What is limbic encephalitis?

Limbic encephalitis is very rare. Approximately 50% of cases occur in patients known to have cancer; in the other 50% the limbic encephalitis is the initial problem. The typical presentation is of a profound amnesic syndrome, without other cognitive problems, often coming on over a few days (occasionally overnight with a stroke-like onset). It progresses rapidly for a period of weeks or months and then seems to stabilize. On examination, patients might have evidence of the primary tumour (most commonly lung cancer but it can be breast or ovarian cancer, lymphoma or other type of tumour). Patients have a profound amnesia but do not have word-finding difficulty. They might show features of other paraneoplastic syndromes, such as a cerebellar syndrome. MRI scanning often shows a high signal in the medial temporal lobes and examination of the CSF classically shows a few lymphocytes and oligoclonal bands. Serological tests are usually positive for anti-Hu antibodies.

METABOLIC DISORDERS THAT CAUSE DEMENTIA

14.24 Many forms of dementia are caused by inborn errors of metabolism present in children. Which of these can affect adults?

The number of storage and metabolic diseases and other inborn errors of metabolism that can cause cognitive problems is legion. All are very rare in adults but those that can occur in adults include:

- Wilson's disease
- mitochondrial disease
- adrenoleukodystrophy
- Fabry's disease
- Kuf's disease and other forms of cerebral inclusion disease
- Hallervorden–Spatz disease
- Niemann–Pick type C.

Generally these diseases present when patients are in their teens or twenties and become even more rare with increasing age. It is usually apparent which patients presenting with a dementia need investigating for an inborn error of metabolism because they:

- are under 40 years; degenerative dementias are extremely rare at this age
- have clear features of a multisystem disease, with cerebellar or extrapyramidal problems or features such as troublesome seizures.

14.25 What are the features of Wilson's disease?

Wilson's disease is an autonomic recessive disease and one of the more common genetic causes of dementia. It is important to be aware of the disease because it is a treatable condition. The average neurologist will see a couple of new cases in a career.

Wilson's disease can present to a gastroenterologist with liver disease; the typical presentation to a neurologist is in the second decade. There is usually no family history of the disease, although occasionally a sibling or cousin will have it. Patients usually develop normally up until the time the illness manifests. It often presents with an atypical psychosis plus a movement disorder. Patients often see a psychiatrist first because their family complains that they have become withdrawn. Patients have a typical facial expression, with a grimace, and rigid limbs, which make writhing (athetoid) movements. They might have seizures. The pathognomic sign on examination is the presence of a brown ring of pigment in the cornea – the Kayser–Fleischer ring.

Routine blood tests often reveal abnormal liver function tests. The most characteristic biochemical abnormality is a low plasma caeruloplasmin (the copper-carrying protein). This is usually tested with the serum copper. In borderline cases, measurement of 24-hour copper excretion, molecular genetic analysis of the Wilson's disease gene or liver biopsy to look for abnormal copper deposition is needed.

Treatment is not straightforward but Wilson's disease responds to treatment with copper-binding agents such as penicillamine. Starting treatment can be associated with a temporary deterioration and seizures.

Once diagnosed other members of the family should be screened.

MOTOR NEURON DISEASE

14.26 Is motor neuron disease associated with dementia?

Textbooks used to state that motor neuron disease was not associated with dementia, but unfortunately this is not true. Most patients with motor neuron disease have some cognitive changes, which can be picked up by a psychologist but which have little effect on their life. Some develop mild problems and might have a mild personality change, becoming either more 'laid back' or sometimes disinhibited. Some develop a more severe frontotemporal dementia similar to that described in Chapter 12. Some have a nominal aphasia. A few patients who initially develop a very typical FTD (see Chapter 12) later develop the motor features of motor neuron disease.

 PATIENT QUESTIONS

14.27 My husband lost his memory for a few hours last Sunday. He has now recovered but remembers nothing of the episode. Is he developing Alzheimer's disease?

The likely diagnosis is transient global amnesia (TGA), a striking episode that is both common and worrying. Typically, patients wake normally but then become suddenly disorientated during the day, they know who they are and recognize their partner and home surroundings but are unable to lay down new memory traces. They appear agitated and ask the same question over and over again, unable to register the answer. The episode lasts 2–6 hours and patients usually recover gradually. Immediately after the event they lose memory for recent events – often covering the last few weeks. Over the next few days the period of amnesia gradually shrinks but they never recall events that occurred during the short period of disorientation.

Various theories have been proposed for TGA, including a brief epileptic seizure or a ministroke, but neither seems to be the cause. TGA is more common in patients with a history of migraine. Recurrences are rare and there is no increased risk of dementia or stroke.

If they are repeated events, particularly those that occur first thing in the morning, then seizures are more likely.

14.28 I have MS. How likely am I to develop dementia?

Although it is possible to pick-up very subtle changes on complex tests in many patients with MS, the likelihood of you developing dementia is small. Most patients who do develop dementia have very severe physical disabilities as well.

Dementia and alcohol

15

15.1 Is there a dementia associated with alcohol abuse?

Yes, patients with chronic alcohol abuse have a much higher incidence of dementia than other individuals. There has long been a debate as to whether alcohol itself causes the dementia through a direct toxic action or whether the dementia is due to indirect causes. There are certainly a number of potent indirect causes of dementia, which include:

- ■ Wernicke–Korsakoff syndrome: this is a metabolic disease predominantly affecting the midbrain. It is caused by a deficiency of thiamine. The characteristic feature is a difficulty in laying down memory traces for more than a few minutes.
- ■ Repetitive head injury: alcoholics are much more prone to head injuries than the normal population and the effects of multiple head injuries, often with neurosurgical complications such as subdural haematoma, can lead to cognitive problems. Cerebral infections are also more common in alcoholics.
- ■ Epilepsy is common in alcoholics and might contribute to the memory problems.
- ■ Acute intoxication with alcohol can complicate the assessment.

15.2 What is Wernicke's encephalopathy?

Wernicke's encephalopathy is the acute phase of thiamine deficiency. It develops over a few hours. Patients become ataxic and disorientated, and might be hallucinating and tremulous as a result of alcohol withdrawal. On examination, there is nystagmus on lateral gaze and often on upgaze. The ankle jerks are usually absent and there may be signs of heart failure from an associated cardiomyopathy. Other features can include an autonomic neuropathy and truncal ataxia.

Treatment is by intravenous thiamine (in the UK this is usually in the form of a multi B vitamin preparation such as Parbinex), which might reverse the changes. However, within a short time the changes become irreversible and Korsakoff's psychosis results.

15.3 Who develops Wernicke's encephalopathy and when?

Alcoholics are the usual victims. It develops only in individuals with a poor diet. Beer usually contains some thiamine and therefore it is unusual in pure beer drinkers. Thiamine deficiency develops slowly and it usually takes many weeks or months of a poor diet before an individual is at risk of developing Wernicke's. The precipitation of the acute encephalopathy is often by a carbohydrate load. It can therefore occur as an iatrogenic disease in hospital when a chronic alcoholic is admitted with a surgical or medical emergency and treated with intravenous dextrose. It occasionally occurs in other diseases, for example patients with malabsorption syndromes or widespread carcinomatosis.

15.4 What is Korsakoff's psychosis?

Korsakoff's psychosis is the chronic disease that follows Wernicke's encephalopathy. Some neurologists believe it is possible to develop Korsakoff's without the acute stage of Wernicke's and certainly it seems that some individuals develop Korsakoff's as a result of a series of mild episodes of confusion without developing full blown Wernicke's.

In Korsakoff's psychosis there is a problem with the laying down of memory traces in a permanent store. Patients can remember the events of the last few minutes – presumably in a temporary store – but have lost the ability to make memories permanent; longer-term memory is relatively spared. In the most dramatic cases the patient has a reasonably normal memory for events up until the onset of Wernicke's, say in June 1989, but the time between June 1989 and 10 minutes ago is lost. The 10-minute window continually changes with time, so it is possible to introduce yourself to the patient every 30 minutes and always to be regarded as a new person.

Another of the features of Korsakoff's psychosis is confabulation. Patients make up rather grandiose stories, presumably to cover the gaps in their memory. There are more widespread problems in Korsakoff's, with reduced motivation and generalized slowing of intellect similar to a subcortical dementia.

15.5 What other neurological problems do patients with alcohol abuse develop?

Patients with Wernicke–Korsakoff's syndrome usually have evidence of other neurological syndromes associated with alcohol abuse. These can include:

■ Central pontine myelinosis: this is a metabolic problem caused by rapid fluctuations in sodium levels and resulting in demyelination in the pons. The clinical picture in the acute stages is a spastic quadriparesis with eye movement problems and dysphagia. It is often iatrogenic – produced medically by too rapid correction of a low sodium level. It is relatively common in alcoholics and, with time, often improves to a limited extent.
■ Cerebellar atrophy: the predominant problem is an unsteady gait; limb ataxia is usually milder. This clinical picture reflects damage to the vermis of the cerebellum.

■ A predominantly sensory peripheral neuropathy: this predominantly affects the feet and can be asymptomatic or cause numbness and pain. The neuropathy might respond to B vitamins and thiamine supplements.

15.6 What investigations should be done in patients with alcohol-related dementia?

If a patient with an alcohol problem presents with a memory problem then it is easy to regard it as one more toxic manifestation of alcohol. However, alcoholics are more prone to a number of problems that can give rise to cognitive problems, including treatable ones, such as epileptic seizures and subdural haematomas from head injury. It is therefore important to investigate and treat these people as carefully as one would other patients.

It is usually appropriate to order a structural scan – a CT or MRI of the brain. This should be done urgently to exclude a subdural haematoma if there is a rapid progression of the dementia or localizing signs.

The usual metabolic screen should be done as laid out in Q 2.45 and an EEG if there is a history suggestive of seizures.

15.7 What are the usual abnormalities on the ACE and MMSE in alcohol-related dementia?

The usual picture on the MMSE is poor recall of three objects and poor attention on the serial 7s. Patients with Wernicke–Korsakoff syndrome are very poorly orientated to time and place and will often confabulate, confidently giving the wrong answer.

There are similar abnormalities on the ACE, with poor verbal fluencies. Naming and visuospatial skills are usually intact.

15.8 How is alcohol-related dementia treated?

If there is an acute deterioration then parenteral thiamine should be given. This can be followed by thiamine 300 mg orally daily with B vitamin complex strong: two tablets three times daily.

The patient should be counselled to cease drinking and offered appropriate referrals for counselling and help with withdrawal.

Other complications, such as epilepsy, subdural haematomas and head trauma need appropriate management.

Human prion diseases

16

16.1 What are prion diseases?

Creutzfeldt–Jakob disease (CJD) is a very rare form of dementia that was little known even to doctors until the 1960s, when a series of scientific breakthroughs led to it becoming famous as an example of a disease caused by a 'slow virus'. Later it was found to be caused by a protein. It remained little known generally until the outbreak of a related disease – bovine spongiform encephalopathy (BSE) – among cows in the UK. Fears that it might spread to humans through the food chain were realized and led to a human form of bovine spongiform encephalopathy, initially called 'new variant CJD' but later 'variant CJD'. Now, prion diseases are some of the most discussed diseases although, even with the variant cases, they remain extremely rare.

16.2 What is a spongiform encephalopathy?

There are a number of alternative names for the group of diseases that includes CJD, the animal prion diseases and kuru; one such name is 'spongiform encephalopathy'. The word 'spongiform' refers to the appearance of the superficial layers of the brain under the microscope; 'encephalopathy' is used rather than 'dementia' because of the rapid progression of the disease.

Prion diseases can be transmitted from one individual to another. This has led to the alternative name of 'transmissible encephalopathies'.

16.3 What human forms of prion disease are there?

There are various human prion diseases. These can be divided into:

- sporadic forms: these include Creutzfeldt–Jakob disease
- iatrogenic forms: where the disease is passed on accidentally as a result of brain or eye surgery or the inoculation of infected material
- genetic forms: which run in families. All the known inherited forms of prion disease are inherited in an autosomal dominant fashion, with up to half the children affected
- dietary forms: such as kuru and variant CJD.

SPORADIC PRION DISEASE

16.4 What is Creutzfeldt–Jakob disease (CJD)?

CJD is a rapidly progressive form of dementia. It usually starts with forgetfulness, clumsiness or visual hallucinations. It is distinguished from virtually all other forms of dementia by its rapid progression. Patients become visibly worse week by week and usually die of their disease within a few months of the onset of their illness. There are also a number of other distinctive features of the disease – during the course of their illness patients with CJD often become mute, they become very clumsy and their gait becomes unsteady and they develop sudden jerks of their limbs and body – myoclonus.

16.5 Why is it called Creutzfeldt–Jakob disease?

Creutzfeldt and Jakob were German neuropathologists who separately described series of patients with unusual forms of neurodegenerative disease. It seems likely that many of the cases they described in their papers were not cases of CJD – so the disease is misnamed. Jakob is sometimes given pre-eminence and the disease is referred to as Jakob–Creutzfeldt disease.

16.6 What is a typical story for a patient with CJD?

CASE STUDY

Brenda Newton, a 58-year-old schoolteacher failed to come to a preterm meeting at her school. A colleague went to her house and was met by a neighbour who said that she was concerned about Brenda. That Brenda had not been around much over the summer holidays and that she had been behaving oddly; she had even been seen staggering at times. The neighbour suggested that alcohol was the problem. Brenda let them in but was quiet and withdrawn. She would answer questions but not initiate conversation. She was dishevelled and clumsy in her movements and made frequent little jerks. There was no sign of alcohol. Brenda's colleague took her to her GP, who immediately admitted her to the local hospital, from where she was transferred to the local neurology unit. All routine investigations were normal except her EEG, which showed some slowing. Within a month of admission she was bedbound and needed help with all activities of daily living. A brain biopsy was considered but not done and she was transferred to a local nursing home where she died 2 months later of pneumonia.

16.7 How common is CJD?

CJD is very rare, with an incidence of one case per million people. The frequency is very similar throughout most of the world and it is equally common in men and women. It is a disease of late middle age rather than the elderly, although there has always been speculation that cases in the very elderly might be unrecognized.

16.8 What causes CJD?

CJD is caused by the accumulation in the brain of an abnormal form of a normal human protein called prion protein. The function of normal prion protein is not known. The abnormal disease-causing form has a very similar structure to the normal. It has exactly the same amino acid sequence and the only difference is the way the protein is folded after it is manufactured. The subtleness of the change needed to convert normal protein to disease protein is probably crucial in the development of the disease.

16.9   How is CJD diagnosed?

As in much of neurology, no one test can diagnose CJD in life; the most important part in the diagnosis is the recognition of the clinical syndrome. A syndrome of progressive ataxia, dementia and myoclonus worsening over a few weeks is very rare and always suggests possible CJD.

There are a number of alternative diagnoses but many of these are accompanied by abnormalities on brain scans and in the CSF; therefore if brain imaging and other tests are normal CJD becomes the likely diagnosis. A number of tests, including CSF analysis and EEG, can produce positive evidence for CJD or other forms of prion disease. This evidence is generally supportive of the diagnosis but not sensitive or specific enough to be conclusive. The 'more common' diseases that might be mistaken for CJD include dementia with Lewy bodies, paraneoplastic syndromes (see Chapter 14), cerebral vasculitis (see Chapter 4) and Hashimoto's encephalopathy (see Chapter 4).

16.10   What changes are seen in the EEG?

In the early stages of prion disease, the EEG can be normal or show the same kind of diffuse slowing seen in the early stages of Alzheimer's disease. Later in the illness it can show a triphasic wave pattern with a constant interval. These abnormalities are called periodic complexes. In the correct clinical context these periodic complexes can be very useful in the diagnosis. Their absence does not exclude the diagnosis and they are seen in a variety of other conditions, such as encephalitis and severe epilepsy.

The other use of the EEG is in patients with a psychiatric presentation – it is often sufficiently abnormal early in the disease to show that the patient has an organic problem rather than a primarily psychiatric one.

16.11   What are the cerebrospinal fluid changes in CJD?

Routine analysis of the CSF in patients with CJD is typically normal. There are no changes in the protein level and no abnormal cells or oligoclonal bands. The test is important in excluding an alternative diagnosis.

CSF analysis for 14-3-3 protein is positive in most patients with sporadic prion disease and in a minority of other cases of dementia. The presence of 14-3-3 protein is not sufficiently specific or sensitive to make a certain diagnosis of prion disease or to exclude it.

16.12   Is there a role for brain biopsy in the diagnosis of CJD?

A brain biopsy is the most accurate way of diagnosing CJD in life, and is also very useful at excluding other potential causes of the patient's problems.

There are three main drawbacks:

- Brain biopsy is invasive and carries a small risk of causing haemorrhage or other complications. The complication rate varies but is approximately 1–3%.
- Brain biopsy is not always helpful. Frustratingly, the biopsy may show no specific changes and does not help the diagnosis. This is less of a problem in the diagnosis of CJD than in other dementias but still a risk.
- There are risks to the surgeons involved and the pathologists who look at the sample. Disposable instruments are used in suspected cases of prion disease to exclude the possibility of transmitting the disease to other neurosurgical patients.

The decision about proceeding to a brain biopsy needs to be made on an individual basis. If the diagnosis appears virtually certain and the patient is in a poor physical condition then most neurologists would not do a biopsy. If the patient has atypical features and is in a good physical condition then there are strong arguments for a biopsy.

The biopsy is examined for the typical morphological features of CJD, such as the diffuse vacuolization in the cortex, but there are also specific stains for the abnormal prion protein to aid the diagnosis.

16.13 Can CJD be treated?

There are no proven treatments for CJD. However, a number of drugs can interfere with protein/protein interactions and there are now excellent animal models of prion disease using transgenic mice. The future for treatment therefore appears good.

No currently available drugs are likely to help the memory and cerebellar problems. Drugs like clonazepam and valproate can help the myoclonus and many of the drug treatments for behavioural problems might also be helpful.

Patients should remain mobile as long as possible and physiotherapy and personal interaction can help maintain function but, in the face of such a rapidly progressive disease, often little can be done.

16.14 What is the prognosis of CJD?

The prognosis of CJD is very poor and the disease is always fatal. There is steady deterioration and the patient usually dies 3–12 months into the illness; some patients survive for 18 months or more. The life expectancy is longer in patients with genetic forms of the disease. Patients with CJD normally die of pneumonia or the other complications of immobility.

16.15 How can a protein cause a disease?

We are used to diseases being caused by living organisms but there is no reason why a protein should not cause a disease. It is likely that the conformation of the prion protein changes in the cell and that the protein assumes a second shape. Normally, this change is reversible but in the presence of plaques of pathogenic prion protein this second form is deposited and gradually accumulates. The accumulation may interfere with the functioning of the cell.

16.16 What is kuru?

Kuru is a disease of the Fore people, who lived in the highlands of New Guinea and were cannibals – eating the bodies and brains of their men who had been killed in battle. The disease was more common in the women and children and it seems likely that it was transmitted either by eating the brains of other humans or smearing the brain over the eyes and mouth. With the end of cannibalism in the 1950s, kuru became a very rare (but not extinct) disease. It presented from childhood onwards with an unsteady gait, tremors and later dementia. Unsteadiness of gait was a major part of the disease and the progress of the disease was measured by whether the patient could walk or needed one stick or two sticks, and so on.

Kuru might seem to be an obscure disease from a different culture and age but it is important for several reasons, the main one being that it was the first form of prion disease to be shown to be transmissible.

Similarities were noticed between the brains of people who had died of kuru and those who had died of sporadic Creutzfeldt disease and transmission studies in CJD proved that kuru is another form of prion disease.

16.17 Is kuru of any relevance today?

There is now a further reason for studying kuru. An outbreak of prion disease after eating human brains in New Guinea in the 1950s parallels the 1990s outbreak of CJD, which was caused by eating infected cow's brains. In both, young people tended to be affected and also in both the source of the infected prion protein was removed after a period – with the ending of cannibalism and the elimination of bovine spongiform encephalopathy. Occasional new cases of kuru are still reported now – 40 or more years after cannibalism died out – suggesting that variant CJD will be a problem for years to come.

IATROGENIC PRION DISEASE

16.18 What are the iatrogenic forms?

A series of cases of iatrogenic CJD followed transmission from asymptomatic individuals in the long incubation period of prion disease to uninfected individuals via surgical instruments. Transmission occurred when inadequately sterilized (for prion protein) surgical instruments were used on other individuals; the majority of cases followed neurosurgery, a few followed eye surgery.

Another group of iatrogenic cases came from individuals injected with human hormones to treat hormone deficiencies. Until the advent of recombinant DNA technologies, human growth hormone and gonadotrophins used to treat dwarfism and other diseases were collected from human brains. The brains from many individuals were needed to extract the growth hormone and to make a single pool of hormone for injection. The pooling of many brains led to the inclusion of occasional individuals who had died of other causes while in the incubation period for sporadic CJD.

Individuals with iatrogenic CJD generally present with a cerebellar syndrome with gait and limb ataxia; cognitive problems develop later. Patients suffering from iatrogenic CJD have a rapid course, dying within a few months of onset of symptoms.

The inoculation of potentially infected brain tissue now seems reckless but unfortunately the prion protein was not denatured by standard sterilizing techniques of the time. Now the risk of transmission is known, new technologies and disposable instruments have made iatrogenic CJD extemely rare.

INHERITED PRION DISEASES

16.19 What about the inherited forms of prion disease?

These are extremely rare, even compared with sporadic CJD. On average, only two new cases are diagnosed in the UK every year. Many are in families known to carry the disease but some appear *de novo* for reasons not dissimilar to those for Huntington's disease (*see* Q 13.32).

The prion protein gene lies on chromosome 20 and, like virtually all genes, each individual has two copies, one on each chromosome.

Many varieties of inherited prion disease have been described and are associated with about 30 different mutations in the prion protein gene. To some extent these mutations 'breed true' – recognizable features are associated with particular mutations. Many of the familial forms start with slowly progressive gait unsteadiness, which often changes little from year to year. Memory problems tend to be less marked than with sporadic CJD. These forms of inherited prion disease are often accompanied by a particular pathology, with complex plaques in the cerebellum, and are called Gerstmann–Straussler syndrome.

Other forms are much more similar to sporadic CJD and can be indistinguishable clinically. Some of the clinical syndromes are more unusual, such as familial fatal insomnia, in which a dementia is accompanied by sleep disturbance and sudden death.

16.20 How can a disease be inherited and transmissible?

Prion disease is virtually unique in that it is both inherited and transmissible.

Prion protein is a natural human protein and therefore, like all proteins, is coded for by a gene. The normal product of this gene – prion protein – occasionally undergoes a subtle change (mutation) to become infective prion protein. The inherited forms of prion disease are caused by such mutations in the prion protein gene. The mutations are in the germ line, are present in all cells and are passed to the next generation. The inherited forms of prion protein produce a mutant protein that varies in amino acid sequence from the wild-type. The abnormal form of prion protein slowly accumulates in plaques, often concentrated in the thalamus and cerebellum. Some inherited forms of prion disease have been transmitted and therefore must be able to interact with normal prion protein to produce accumulations of abnormal prion protein in a similar fashion to that seen in sporadic prion disease.

16.21 What causes sporadic CJD?

This is not known. The uniform distribution around the world and the lack of a relationship to environmental factors suggest that a change in the prion gene, some time in later life, alters the nature of the prion protein – a so-called somatic mutation. These are not passed on to future generations. There are a number of alternative possibilities, such as a link to the sheep prion disease, scrapie, but little evidence has been found for these.

16.22 What animal forms of prion disease are there?

A large number of animal forms of prion disease have been described. Scrapie is a disease of sheep and there is evidence from fossils that it has been present for centuries. A number of other naturally occurring forms of prion disease have been described. Bovine spongiform encephalopathy (BSE) is a disease of cattle. There was an epidemic of BSE in the UK in the 1980s and 1990s, and it has been recorded in many other countries subsequently. Many thousands of cattle were infected with BSE and many entered the human food chain and were also fed to domestic and zoo animals. This led to a series of novel prion diseases, including variant CJD.

16.23 Where did BSE come from?

This has been a much-debated topic. Its source is not clear and many theories have been expounded. There is not much evidence to link it with the much longer-established disease of sheep, scrapie. However, once BSE was established in the UK beef herd it seems beyond doubt that the process of feeding the remains of one generation of cattle to the next via processed cattle meal led to the epidemic. This process of commercial cannibalism had taken place for many years but high temperatures used to be employed in the rendering process so that tallow could be produced for the candle industry. The temperature used to extract tallow was sufficiently high to destroy the prion protein. The fall in the demand for tallow led to a lowering of the temperature used to render carcasses, this resulted in the survival of the BSE agent in the feed and allowed for the rapid and widespread dissemination of the disease throughout the dairy and beef herds.

16.24 Is variant CJD the human form of BSE?

The question of whether human variant CJD (vCJD) is a result of the BSE epidemic is clearly of great public health interest. The appearance of an apparently novel prion disease a few years after the peak of the BSE epidemic is clearly worrying (all human prion diseases have an incubation period of years). There is now good evidence to suggest that vCJD is the human form of BSE. The most important and direct evidence comes from animal experiments – prion diseases can be transmitted to laboratory transgenic animals (animals containing genes from other species) and the prion protein isolated from the brains of these animals retains features of the original infecting prion protein. In other words, strains of prion protein can run true despite transmission to other species. The characteristics of the strain of prion protein isolated from human victims of vCJD and transmitted to transgenic animals are very similar to those isolated from the brains of cows with BSE, thus confirming the common ancestry of the two diseases.

So far, vCJD has occurred only in individuals with a genotype that has sequences that code for the amino acid methionine at codon 129 in both prion genes.

16.25 How does vCJD present?

The symptoms of vCJD are rather different from sporadic CJD and, in retrospect, rather distinctive. However, the early symptoms are shared by many more common diseases. The first problems – depression and anxiety – tend to lead to referral to a psychiatrist. The depression might be accompanied by painful sensory symptoms in the limbs and face. This phase can last for several months without clear progression of the problems. Then the patient enters the phase with clear neurological problems, with a combination of a cerebellar, thalamic and cerebral problems. The patient's walking becomes less steady, the arms become clumsy and myoclonus develops. A number of patients will develop chorea – a more continuous jerky movement of the limbs. Patients become withdrawn, their personality changes and they develop cognitive problems. The course of variant disease is typically longer than sporadic CJD. It is universally fatal and most patients die between 1 and 2 years from the onset of the disease.

16.26 What does examination reveal in vCJD?

In the early stages of vCJD, when the patient has a mood disturbance and sensory symptoms, the neurological examination is probably normal. However, physical signs are usually present in the neurological phase of the disease. These start with gait disturbance and clumsiness of the limbs. Myoclonus of limbs or trunk is often present. Some individuals develop a florid movement disorder with chorea; others show signs of brainstem disease, such as a supranuclear gaze palsy. The cognitive problems are usually frontal in nature with poor attention and concentration combined with a paucity of spontaneous speech. As the disease progresses, more florid cerebellar and pyramidal problems develop and patients become bed-bound, with a spastic quadraparesis.

16.27 Can vCJD be passed on through blood transfusion or surgery?

Prion protein accumulates in lymphoid cells and tissue before producing symptoms. Theoretically, therefore, vCJD can be passed on through blood transfusion or surgery involving lymphoid tissue (including appendicectomy and tonsillectomy). This is being closely monitored. So far, there is no evidence for transmission. However, prion protein has been detected in one routine surgical sample (of thousands tested).

16.28 Are there any treatments for vCJD?

Despite the recent publicity there is no proven treatment for vCJD. However, a number of drugs might work and clinical trials are currently taking place. Quinacrine and chlorpromazine have been suggested as treatments. Trials of quinacrine are underway at present. The use of chlorpromazine is limited by the side-effects it produces in patients with dementia.

16.29 How can vCJD be diagnosed?

The diagnosis in the early stages is very difficult and it is unreasonable to expect doctors to pick out the very rare cases of vCJD from the myriad of patients with depression and sensory symptoms. By the time it is clear that memory and balance are affected the diagnosis usually becomes clear. Tests that can be helpful in sporadic CJD, such as EEG and 14-3-3 protein analysis of the CSF, are much less useful in vCJD.

The MRI scan has a characteristic appearance, with high signal, particularly on FLAIR images in the posterior part of the thalamus (the pulvinar). If the diagnosis remains unclear, biopsy of the tonsils detects the abnormal prion protein with very high sensitivity and specificity.

 PATIENT QUESTIONS

16.30 How many cases of vCJD will there be?

This is a difficult question. At the current time there have been 127 cases in the UK and a handful of cases in other countries (especially France and Japan). From time to time there is a report that the estimates have been revised up or down by the experts but the truth is that we do not have enough information to give an accurate estimate. This is not to criticize those whose job it is to predict the unpredictable. As time goes by and the annual rate remains at about 20 cases a year we can breathe a bit more easily as the odds on an outbreak involving tens of thousands of cases become a little longer. However, there are still new cases of kuru 40 or more years after the source (cannibalism) died out, so it will be many years before vCJD disappears.

16.31 My husband has developed CJD. How much does he know?

CJD and vCJD are terrible diseases in which the affected individual deteriorates rapidly. In the very early stages of the disease the sufferer is often aware of problems, although they tend to underestimate them. In the middle and later stages of the disease the majority of patients have little or no insight into their problems – they are unaware of what is happening to them.

16.32 Is there a support organization for patients and relatives affected by vCJD?

Yes, there is a very active group that has fought very hard to publicize the fate of individuals infected by this terrible disease. It played a major role in obtaining compensation from the government for victims and will provide information and help (www.hbsef.org.uk).

GLOSSARY

ACE	Addenbrookes Cognitive Examination	**HAART**	highly active antiretroviral therapy
ACh	acetylcholine	**HIV**	human immunodeficiency virus
AChEI	acetylcholine-esterase inhibitor	**ICD**	International Classification of Diseases
AD	Alzheimer's disease		
ADI	Alzheimer's Disease International	**IV**	intravenous
ADL	activities of daily living	**LBD**	Lewy body disease
Aids	acquired immunodeficiency syndrome	**LFT**	liver function tests
		MAOI	monoamine oxidase inhibitor
ANCA	antineutrophil cytoplasmic antibodies	**MCI**	mild cognitive impairment
		MHA	Mental Health Act
apo E	apoliopoprotein E	**MID**	multi-infarct dementia
APP	amyloid precursor protein	**MMSE**	Mini Mental State Examination
AS	Alzheimer's Society	**MRI**	magnetic resonance imaging
BSE	bovine spongiform encephalopathy	**MS**	multiple sclerosis
		MSU	midstream urine
CADASIL	cerebral autosomal dominant arteriopathy with subcortical ischaemic leukoencephalopathy	**MTS**	Mental Test Score
		NICE	National Institute for Clinical Excellence
		NMDA	N-methyl-d-aspartate
CBD	corticobasal degeneration	**NPH**	normal pressure hydrocephalus
CJD	Creutzfeldt–Jakob disease		
CNS	central nervous system	**OT**	occupational therapist
CPN	community psychiatric nurse	**PEG**	percutaneous gastrostomy
CRP	C-reactive protein	**PET**	positron emission tomography
CSF	cerebrospinal fluid	**PML**	progressive multifocal leukoencephalopathy
CT	computerized tomography		
CXR	chest X-ray	**PS1/PS2**	presenilin (genes 1 and 2)
DLB	dementia with Lewy bodies	**PSP**	progressive supranuclear palsy
DLB/PD	dementia with Lewy bodies/Parkinson's disease	**SDAT**	senile dementia Alzheimer type
		SPECT	single photon emission computed tomography
DVLA	Driver and Vehicle Licensing Agency		
		SSRI	selective serotonin reuptake inhibitor
ECG	electrocardiogram		
EEG	electroencephalogram	**TCA**	tricyclic antidepressant
EMI	elderly mentally infirm	**TFT**	thyroid function tests
EPoA	enduring power of attorney	**TPHA**	*Trepenoma pallidum* haemagglutination
ESR	erythrocyte sedimentation rate		
FBC	full blood count	**U&E**	urea and electrolytes
FTA	fixed trepenome haemagglutination	**VaD**	vascular dementia
		vCJD	variant Creutzfeldt-Jakob disease
FTD	frontotemporal dementia		
GP	general practitioner	**VDRL**	Venereal Disease Reference Laboratory
H&E	haematoxylin and eosin		

APPENDIX 1
The Addenbrooke's Cognitive Examination (ACE)

ADDENBROOKE'S COGNITIVE EXAMINATION (ACE)

ADDENBROOKE'S / NORFOLK & NORWICH DEPARTMENTS OF NEUROLOGY

Name :	Age at leaving education : _____
Date of birth :	*(school/college etc.)*
Hospital no. :	Date of testing : ---- / ---- / ----
Addressograph	Tester's name : --------------------

ORIENTATION

(a) What is the
Year ------------------
Season ------------------
Date ±2 ------------------
Record Day ------------------
errors. Month ------------------

(b) Where are we
Country ------------------
County ------------------
Town ------------------
Record Hospital/building ------------------
errors. Floor *Allow if almost correct.* ------------------

[*Score 0–5*]

[*Score 0–5*]

REGISTRATION

Name three unrelated objects, taking one second to say each: e.g. **lemon, key & ball.** Say them once only and ask the patient to repeat all three. *Give one point for each correct answer at first attempt.*
If score <3 repeat the items until the patient learns all 3.

[0–3]

ATTENTION/CONCENTRATION

Ask the patient to **begin with 100 and subtract 7, and keep subtracting 7.**
Stop after five subtractions (93, 86, 79, 72, 65). *Score the total number of correct subtractions. If score <5:* Spell **WORLD backwards.** *Score is the number of letters in the correct order, eg.dlorw = 3.*
Take score of better of the two tasks. Record errors: --------------------------

[0–5]

RECALL Ask for the names of the 3 objects learned in question 3. *One point for each answer.*

[0–3]

MEMORY

(a) **Anterograde Memory:**
Read the name and address and ask the patient to repeat it once you have finished.
Regardless of the score after the first trial, repeat the task twice in exactly the same way.
Record errors at each trial.

	1st trial	2nd	3rd	5 min delay			
Peter Marshall	--- ---	--- ---	--- ---	--- ---			
42 Market Street	--- --- ---	--- --- ---	--- --- ---	--- --- ---			
Chelmsford	---	---	---	---			
Essex	---	---	---	---	Trial 1–3	[0–21]	
	/7	/7	/7	/7	5 min delay	[0–7]	

(b) **Retrograde Memory:**

Record errors.

Name of PM	--------------------
Last PM	--------------------
Opposition Leader	--------------------
USA President	--------------------

[0–4]

VERBAL FLUENCY

(a) **Letters**   Ask the patient to generate as many words as possible beginning with the letter **P** in one minute; proper nouns (people and places etc.) are not allowed.

(b) **Animals**   In the same way ask the patient to generate the names of as many animals as possible in one minute; beginning with **any letter of the alphabet**.

Record all responses. Error types: perseverations and intrusions

	P			Animals	
(*start here*)	(*continue*)		(*start here*)	(*continue*)	

Animal	P	Score
>21	>17	7
17–21	14–17	6
14–16	11–13	5
11–13	8–10	4
9–10	6–7	3
7–8	4–5	2
<7	<4	1

P   :   Total _____   No. correct _____   [0–7] ☐
Animals: Total _____   No. correct _____   [0–7] ☐

LANGUAGE

(a) **Spontaneous speech**   • fluency (phrases <5 words)
    Describe only   • paraphasic errors (phonemic or semantic)
    Do NOT score   • word finding difficulties

(b) **Naming**   Ask the patient to name the following pictures   [0–2] ☐
                           Record errors

                                                            [0–10] ☐

(c) **Comprehension**	Single-step commands	
	• "point to the door"	[0–2]
	• "point to the ceiling"	[0–1]
	• show written instruction:	

CLOSE YOUR EYES

	3-stage command	
	• "Take the paper in your hand.	
	Fold the paper in half.	
	Put the paper on the floor."	
	Score 1 for each correctly performed step.	[0–3]

	Complex grammar	
	• "point to the ceiling then the door"	
	• "point to the door after touching the bed/desk"	
	Score 1 for each correctly performed command.	[0–2]

(d) **Repetition**	single words	
	• "brown"	
	• "conversation"	
	• "articulate"	[0–3]

	phrases	
	• "No ifs, ands, or buts"	[0–1]
	• "The orchestra played and the	
	audience applauded."	[0–1]

(e) **Reading**	• shed	
	• wipe	
	• board	
	• flame	
	• bridge *Score 1 if all regular words correct.*	[0–1]
	• sew	
	• pint	
	• soot	
	• dough	
	• height *Score 1 if all irregular words correct.*	[0–1]

(f) **Writing**	Ask the patient to **make up a sentence and write it down** in the space below. If stuck, suggest a topic e.g. weather, journey to hospital. *Score 1 for a correct subject and verb in a meaningful sentence.*	
		[0–1]

_____

NOW CHECK delayed recall of name and address. Record errors on page 1 and enter result into box.

VISUOSPATIAL ABILITIES

(a) **Overlapping pentagons**   Ask the patient to copy this diagram:

Score 1 if both figures have 5 sides and overlap.   [0–1]

(b) **Wire cube**   Ask the patient to copy this drawing:

Score 1 if correct   [0–1]

(c) **Clock**   Ask the patient to draw a clockface with numbers and the hands at ten past five

Score 1 each for correct circle, numbers and hands. [0–3]

CHECK: *Have you tested and recorded the delayed recall of name and address (page 1)?*

OVERALL SCORES   **TOTAL:**   **/100**

MDP/Version 2/1999

Normative values based on 127 controls aged 50–80.
Mean 93.8 ± 3.5   Cut off < 88 gives 93% sensitivity 71% specificity for dementia
Cut off < 83 gives 82% sensitivity 96% specificity for dementia

APPENDIX 2
Drugs used in the treatment of dementia

This list is not intended to be comprehensive. It includes a selection of the most commonly prescribed drugs in patients with dementia, associated psychiatric disorders and Parkinson's disease. Where there are several drugs in one class with similar characteristics, only examples are listed.

This appendix is not intended to be a guide to prescribing.

AMANTIDINE

A very long established drug for Parkinson's disease. It is sometimes used early in the disease but is increasingly used to treat patients suffering with fluctuations in disability late in the disease. It can cause a leg rash and hallucinations.

APOMORPHINE

Apomorphine is a dopamine agonist that can be given by subcutaneous injection for quick action or by continuous infusion in patients with advanced Parkinson's disease. It is usually given with domperidone to counter the nausea it produces.

B VITAMINS COMPLEX STRONG

Used as an adjunct to thiamine in alcohol-related dementia. The usual course is two tablets tds for a month.

BENZHEXOL

Anticholinergic. Used to reduce the tremor in Parkinson's disease. The starting dose is 0.5 mg bd increased up to 4 mg bd. It can worsen confusion and therefore is little used in dementia with Lewy bodies.

CARBAMAZEPINE

Anticonvulsant. The first choice drug in focal epilepsy (which is virtually all epilepsy with onset after the age of 25 years). Useful for treating seizures secondary to Alzheimer's disease and other dementias. Also the drug to use in patients who present with memory problems due to seizures. The starting dose is 100 mg bd, increasing over a month to 400 mg bd. The maximum dose in most people is 1600 mg – 2 g per day. It always causes side-effects at the start of treatment (diplopia, drowsiness, unsteadiness) but these virtually always settle over a couple of weeks.

CLONAZEPAM

Benzodiazepine. Reduces myoclonus in degenerative dementias. The starting dose is usually 0.5 mg once daily and the maximum dose usually 2 mg bd. It can cause sedation and can be addictive.

CORTICOSTEROIDS

Many uses in neurological disease, including the treatment of MS relapses and cerebral vasculitis.

DONEZEPIL (ARICEPT)

Cholinesterase inhibitor. Licensed for use in mild to moderate Alzheimer's disease. Also reported to be effective in dementia with Lewy bodies. The starting dose is 5 mg daily taken in the evening usually; maximum dose is 10 mg.

DOPAMINE AGONISTS

These drugs act directly on the dopamine receptors and help alleviate the motor problems of Parkinson's disease. They are often used as first-line treatment in early disease in younger patients and as add-on treatment to L-dopa in patients established on Sinemet or Madopar.

Various dopamine agonists are now used. They can all cause nausea (usually controllable with the addition of domperidone), and they can also cause hallucinations, low blood pressure, confusion and drowsiness.

The major dopamine agonists used at present are cabergoline, pergolide, pramipexole and ropinorole.

Cabergoline

A dopamine agonist with the advantage of a long halflife and can therefore be given once a day. A typical starting dose is 0.5 mg once daily building up to 4–6 mg once a day.

Pergolide

A longer established dopamine agonist that is given at a starting dose of 50 micrograms daily, building up to 1mg three times a day

Pramipexole

A dopamine agonist that is marketed as having a larger effect on tremor than other dopamine agonists. It is started at a dose of 125 micrograms three times daily, building up to 0.5 mg three times a day.

Ropinorole

A dopamine agonist used to treat Parkinson's disease. A typical starting dose is 0.25 mg three times a day increasing gradually to 4–6 mg three times a day.

ENTACAPONE

This drug has no anti-Parkinson's action of its own but inhibits L-dopa metabolism. It is used to prolong the action of L-dopa; 200 mg is given with each L-dopa dose (up to eight times a day).

FLUOXETINE

Selective serotonin reuptake inhibitor (SSRI) – an antidepressant. It has a low side-effect profile and is therefore a useful drug in patients with both depression and dementia. It appears to have a selective action (together with the other SSRIs) in treating some behavioural problems in FTD, for example the overeating and the stereotyped regimes. The starting dose is 20 mg daily, this may need to be doubled. Other examples of SSRIs include citalopram, paroxetine, sertraline and fluvoxamine.

GALANTAMINE (REMINYL)

Cholinesterase inhibitor. Licensed for use in mild to moderate Alzheimer's disease. Also thought to be effective in dementia with Lewy bodies. The starting dose is 4 mg twice daily for 4 weeks increasing to 8 mg twice daily for 4 weeks. Maintenance dose is 8–12 mg twice daily.

HALOPERIDOL

Conventional neuroleptic. Licensed for psychotic disorders and mania. Used in low doses (0.50–1.5 mg daily) for agitation in dementia. But extrapyramidal side-effects are often troublesome.

MADOPAR

A drug that combines L-dopa – the precursor of dopamine – with a drug that prevents its breakdown outside the brain. It is one of the mainstays of treatment of Parkinson's disease. A typical starting dose is 62.5 mg three times a day increasing over a month to 125 mg three times a day. Madopar comes in a variety of preparations, including slow-release forms and dispersible forms for slow sustained and quick action, respectively. Side-effects include nausea (which can be prevented by adding domperidone) and hallucinations

MEMANTINE (EBIXA)

Glutamatergic modulator. Licensed for use in moderate to severe Alzheimer's disease. Also reported to be effective in vascular dementia. The starting dose is 5 mg daily increasing by 5 mg every week until the maintenance dose of 20 mg daily is achieved.

OLANZAPINE (ZYPREXIA)

Atypical neuroleptic. Licensed for schizophrenia but in low doses (2.5–10 mg) used for behavioural problems in dementia. Has fewer extrapyramidal side-effects than older neuroleptics.

PARENTEROVITE

Proprietary preparation of B vitamins, including thiamine, which is used to treat acute Wernicke's syndrome. Given parenterally (usually slow intravenous infusion). There is a risk of anaphylaxis but it should be given in the acute situation if Wernicke's is suspected to prevent the later disabling Korsakoff's psychosis, which is untreatable. Usually given daily for 3 days and then followed by 1-month course of oral thiamine and B vitamin complex strong as outlined above.

QUETIAPINE (SEROQUEL)

Atypical neuroleptic. Licensed for schizophrenia. In low doses (25–50 mg daily) useful for behavioural problems in patients with dementia. Experience so far suggests that extrapyramidal side-effects are rare.

RISPERIDONE (RISPERDAL)

Atypical neuroleptic. Licensed for schizophrenia but in low doses (0.5–2.0 mg daily) used for behavioural problems in dementia. Has fewer extrapyramidal side-effects than conventional neuroleptics but at higher doses these can still be troublesome.

RIVASTIGMINE (EXELON)

Cholinesterase inhibitor. Licensed for use in mild to moderate Alzheimer's disease. Also reported to be effective in dementia with Lewy bodies. The starting dose is 1.5 mg twice daily increased every 4 weeks in aliquots of 3 mg daily to a maximum dose of 6 mg bd.

SELEGILENE

A drug that has fluctuated in popularity. It was used primarily as the first-line treatment but is now used later in the course of the disease. It does not have a powerful effect.

SINEMET

A drug that combines L-dopa – the precursor of dopamine – with a drug that prevents its breakdown outside the brain. It differs from Madopar in the peripheral inhibitor included. Sinemet is one of the mainstays of treatment of Parkinson's disease. A typical starting dose is Sinemet ls, one tablet three times a day increasing over a month, to Sinemet 110, one tablet three times a day. It comes in a variety of preparations, including slow-release forms for slow sustained action. Side-effects include nausea (which can be prevented by adding domperidone) and hallucinations.

SULPIRIDE

Conventional neuroleptic. Useful for behavioural problems in dementia and also for reducing abnormal movements, such as the chorea in

Huntington's disease. The starting dose is usually 200 mg daily increasing to 300 mg bd.

TETRABENAZINE

Modulates dopamine transmission. Reduces the chorea in Huntington's disease. Its use is often limited by its side-effects, which include depression.

THIAMINE

B group vitamin. Used to treat chronic memory problems in alcohol-related dementia. The usual course is 300 mg daily for a month.

VALPROATE

Anticonvulsant. Can be effective for the myoclonus and seizures seen in degenerative dementias. The starting dose is 200 mg tds increasing to 500 mg bd.

VENLAFAXINE

Serotonin and noradrenaline reuptake inhibitor (SNRI) – an antidepressant. Also licensed for generalized anxiety. Quite well tolerated in the elderly. Dose range 75–225 mg daily.

ACTION ON ELDER ABUSE

Astral House, 1268 London Road, London SW16 4ER
Tel: 0808 808 8141 (helpline)/020 8764 7648 (admin)
www.freespace.virgin.net/man.web/aea/
Offers emotional support in a wide range of languages. It aims to prevent emotional, physical, sexual and financial abuse of older people by raising awareness.

AGE CONCERN

Astral House, 1268 London Road, London SW16 4ER
Tel: 020 8765 7200
www.ageconcern.org.uk
Provides advice for patients and carers and help in locating local support groups and services, including day centres, lunch clubs, home visits and transport services.

THE ALZHEIMER'S SOCIETY

Gordon House, 10 Greencoat Place, London SW1P 1PH
Tel: 020 7306 0606
Fax: 020 7306 0808
e-mail: enquiries@alzheimers.org.uk
www.alzheimers.org.uk/
Leading care and research charity in England, Wales and Northern Ireland for people with all forms of dementia and their carers. Produces information, advice and fact sheets on many different topics, and runs a network of carers groups, carers contacts, befriending projects and telephone helplines.

ALZHEIMER SCOTLAND

Alzheimer Scotland – Action on Dementia, 22 Drumsheugh Gardens, Edinburgh EH3 7RN
Tel: 0131 243 1453
Fax: 0131 243 1450
e-mail: alzheimer@alzscot.org
www.alzscot.org/index.html
Scotland's leading dementia charity. Provides information and services such as advocacy, drop-in centres and home support. Campaigns to help people

with dementia and their families and carers. The website includes dementia information in a range of languages including Bengali, Chinese, Hindi, Urdu and Polish.

ALZHEIMER'S SOCIETY OF IRELAND

43 Northumberland Avenue, Dun Laoghaire, Co. Dublin, Ireland
Tel: 00 353 1 284 6616
Gives support to families and provides information on Alzheimer's Disease and dementia.

THE BSE INQUIRY

www.bse.org.uk
The official site for the Bovine Spongiform Encephalopathy Inquiry.

HUMAN BSE FOUNDATION

www.hbsef.org
Set up and run by families who have lost loved ones to variant Creutzfeldt-Jakob disease.

CJD SUPPORT NETWORK

Helpline 01630 673 973
www.alzheimers.org.uk/cjd/index.html
Linked to the Alzheimer's Society. Focused on providing practical support and information about all forms of CJD to professionals, families and patients, promoting research into CJD and lobbying government.

CJD INFORMATION AND GUIDANCE

www.doh.gov.uk/cjd/cjdl
www.doh.gov.uk/cjd/cjdguidance

THE UK CREUTZFELDT–JAKOB DISEASE SURVEILLANCE UNIT

www.cjd.ed.ac.uk

CANDID (COUNSELLING AND DIAGNOSIS IN DEMENTIA)

Box 16, The National Hospital for Neurology and Neurosurgery, Queen Square, London WC1N 3BG
Tel: 020 7829 8773
e-mail: research@dementia.ion.ucl.ac.uk
www.candid.ion.ucl.ac.uk
CANDID and The Dementia Research Group based at the National Hospital for Neurology and Neurosurgery provide a clinical assessment and diagnosis facility under the NHS for UK residents (GP referral required), fact sheets on dementia and prion disease, and links to journal articles.

CARERS NATIONAL

Tel: 020 7490 8818

CARERS UK

Tel 0808 808 777 (10 a.m. to noon and 2 to 4 p.m)
www.carersuk.demon.uk
Local branch information is given on the website.

CARING MATTERS

132 Gloucester Place, London NW1 6DT
Tel: 020 7402 2702
e-mail: info@caring-matters.org.uk
www.caring-matters.org.uk
Information for carers in the UK, covering topics such as advocacy, financial and legal matters, selecting home help or care homes, coping with caring.

COUNSEL AND CARE

Twyman House, 16 Bonny Street, London NW1 9PG
Tel: 020 7485 1550 (9.30 a.m. to 4.30 p.m.)
e-mail: counsel&care@counselandcare.demon.co.uk
www.charitynet.org/%7Ecounsel+care/
National advice and information service for older people, their carers, relatives and professionals working with them. Advice via telephone and letter on a wide range of subjects such as welfare benefits, accommodation, residential care, community care and hospital discharge. Also practical help (advocacy and grants) and fact sheets.

CROSSROADS

10 Regent Place, Rugby, Warwickshire CV21 2PN
Tel: 01788 573653
www.crossroads.org.uk
The Crossroads scheme 'Caring for Carers' has over 200 schemes across England and Wales providing carers with high-quality support. Trained careworkers go into the home and take over the caring tasks, enabling the carer to go shopping, have some free time or even catch up with sleep.

CENTRE FOR POLICY ON AGEING

Tel: 020 7253 1787
www.cpa.org.uk
Promotes informed debate about issues affecting older age groups, stimulates awareness of the needs of older people and encourages good practice. Primarily directed towards informing and influencing service providers.

DEMENTIA CARE TRUST

Kingsley House, Greenbank Road, Bristol BS5 6HE

Tel: 0870 443 5325

Fax: 0117 951 8213

www.dct.org.uk

Provides relief caring at home, counselling and day care. Based in Bristol but expanding its coverage.

THE DEMENTIA RELIEF TRUST

6 Camden High Street, London NW1 0JH

Tel: 020 7874 7210

Fax: 020 7874 7219

www.dementiarelief.org.uk

Aims to improve the quality of life for people with dementia and their carers. Offers training for carers of the elderly and training, support and promotion of the Admiral Nurse initiative.

EAC HOUSING CARE

3rd Floor, 89 Albert Embankment, London SE1 7PT

Tel: 020 7820 1343

Fax: 020 7820 3970

e-mail: enquiries@e-a-c.demon.co.uk

www.housingcare.org

Infomation, resources and links for sheltered and retirement housing, and residential care.

HELP THE AGED

207–221 Pentonville Road, London N1 9UZ

Tel: 020 7278 1114

Senior line: 0808 800 6565 (weekdays 9 a.m. to 4 p.m.) for free welfare rights advice.

Fax: 020 7278 1116

e-mail: info@helptheaged.org.uk

www.helptheaged.org.uk

Provides practical support to help older people live independent lives.

PARKINSON'S DISEASE SOCIETY OF THE UNITED KINGDOM

215 Vauxhall Bridge Road, London SW1V 1EJ

Helpline: 0808 800 0303

www.parkinsons.org.uk

The Parkinson's Disease Society is the UK support group for patients with Parkinson's disease. The PDS website gives basic information about the disease and is written in simple terms to help patients to understand. The website also provides news about the disease and details of how to join or contact the PDS.

PICK'S DISEASE SUPPORT GROUP

Tel 0116 271 1414
e-mail carol@pdsg.org.uk
www.pdsg.org.uk
Provides information and advice for carers of patients with frontotemporal dementia, Pick's disease, frontal lobe degeneration, dementia with Lewy bodies, corticobasal degeneration and alcohol-related dementia.

THE PRINCESS ROYAL TRUST FOR CARERS

Tel 020 7480 7788
e-mail prt4c@aol.com
www.carers.org
A network of carers centres, providing information, support services and practical help.

THE RELATIVES AND RESIDENTS ASSOCIATION

Tel: 020 7916 6055
Provides help and advice for people in long-term care facilities.

SOLICITORS FOR THE ELDERLY (SFE)

www.solicitorsfortheelderly.com
An interest group led by solicitors for practitioners providing a comprehensive range of high-quality legal services for older people, their family and carers.

THE STROKE ASSOCIATION

Stroke House, 123–127 Whitecross Street, London EC1Y 8JJ
Tel: 020 7566 0300
www.stroke.org.uk
National organization providing practical support – including telephone helplines, publications and welfare grants – to people who have had strokes, their families and carers. At local levels, the Stroke Association provides family support workers and a community service called Dysphasia Support – volunteers work to improve communication skills with people who have lost the ability to speak, read or write.

OTHER RELEVANT WEBSITES

These websites were verified before publication but some might have closed down since. It is important to note that not all sites are regularly updated.

www.age2000.org.uk
The website for the Debate of the Age is a useful resource for those interested in the political and social aspects of ageing.

www.alzheimers.org.uk
The Alzheimer's Society website is an important resource for professionals, patients and carers with much information and advice on dementia care.

www.alz.co.uk
Alzheimer's Disease International promotes dementia research and services in the developing world. This site also provides useful information for carers.

www.alzforum.org
The Alzheimer Research Forum. An 'on-line scientific community'. Current and 'milestone' scientific papers, news on research developments.

www.alzheimer.ca
The website of the Alzheimer's Association (Canada).

www.alz.org
The website of the Alzheimer's Association (USA).

www.alznsw.asn.au
The website of the Alzheimer's Association of New South Wales (Australia).

www.alzvic.asn.au/index
The website of the Alzheimer's Association of Victoria (Australia).

www.bgs.org.uk
The official website of the British Geriatrics Society. It includes useful links to geriatric societies in other countries.

www.bmj.com/cgi/collection/dementia
A collection of articles on dementia from the *British Medical Journal*.

www.dementia.ion.ucl.ac.uk
Website of the Dementia Research Group. It includes details of ongoing research – with excellent images – and information on young-onset dementia and the genetics of dementia. There is also a link to the CANDID website, which contains fact sheets.

www.healthandage.com
US-based website. News, articles and FAQs on dementia. Also links to other sites. Funded by the pharmaceutical industry.

www.hebs.scot.nhs.uk/topics/topictitles.cfm?topic=mental
Health Education Board for Scotland (HEBS) patient information booklet for patients diagnosed with dementia.

www.ipa-online.org
The website of the International Psychogeriatric Association offers extensive links and educational material.

www.memoryzine.com
The website of the US-based Practical Memory Institute.

www.ccc.nottingham.ac.uk/~mpzjlowe/lewy/lewyhome
LEWYNET is primarily concerned with dementia with Lewy bodies but also includes pages on other dementias and links to other sites.

www.open.gov.uk
The place to go for policy documents and governmental reports.

www.parkinsonsdisease.com
Access to information for primary-care physicians, patients and specialists. Addresses and contact details of support groups are listed by country. FAQs from patients and articles written by patients with young-onset PD.

www.pdsg.org.uk
Website for carers of patients with frontal lobe dementias and dementia with Lewy bodies. Newsletters, articles, forum, details of meetings.

www.rcpsych.ac.uk
The website of the Royal College of Psychiatrists (UK) includes a link to *Old Age Psychiatrist*, the quarterly publication of the Faculty of Old Age. This publishes articles on a wide variety of topics, many related to dementia and of interest to a multidisciplinary readership.

www.dvla.gov.uk
The website for the Driver and Vehicle Licensing Agency. It provides information on the legal aspects of driving with dementia.

SELECTED REFERENCES AND FURTHER READING

Beattie A, Daker-White G, Gilliard J, Means R 2002 Younger people in dementia care. A review of service needs, service provision and models of good practice. Aging and Mental Health 6(3):205–212

Burns A, Jacoby R, Levy R 1990 Psychiatric phenomena in Alzheimer's Disease. British Journal of Psychiatry 157:72–94

Burns A, Zaudig M 2002 Mild cognitive impairment in older people. Lancet 360:1963–1965

Dunkin J, Anderson-Hanley C 1998 Dementia care-giver burden: a review of the literature and guidelines for assessment and intervention. Neurology 51(Suppl 1):S53–S60

Folstein M, Folstein S, McHugh P 1975 Mini Mental State: a practical method for grading the cognitive state of patients for clinicians. Journal of Psychiatric Research 12:189–198

Greenfield S 1998 Brain drugs of the future. British Medical Journal 317:1698–1701

Hachinski V, Iliff L, Zilkha E et al 1975 Cerebral blood flow in dementia. Archives of Neurology 32:632–637

Hodgkinson H 1972 Evaluation of a mental test score (MTS) for assessment of mental impairment in the elderly. Age and Aging 1:223–230

International Psychogeriatric Association 1996 Behavioural and psychological signs and symptoms of dementia (BPSD). Implications for research and treatment. International Psychogeriatrics 8:Suppl 3

Lund and Manchester Group 1994 Clinical and neuropathological criteria for fronto-temporal dementia. Journal of Neurology and Neurosurgical Psychology 57:416–418

McKeith I, Galasko D, Kosaka K et al 1996 Consensus guidelines for the clinical and pathologic diagnosis of dementia with Lewy bodies (DLB); report of the Consortium on DLB International Workshop. Neurology 47:1113–1124

McKhann G, Drachman D, Folstein M et al 1984 Clinical diagnosis of Alzheimer's disease. Neurology 34:939–944

O'Brien J, Ballard C 2001 Drugs for Alzheimer's disease. British Medical Journal 323:123–124

Ritchie K, Lovestone S 2002 The dementias. Lancet:360 1759–1766

Rocca A, Hofman A, Brayne C et al 1991 Frequency and distribution of Alzheimer's disease in Europe. Annals of Neurology 30:381–390

Skoog I 1998 Status of risk factors for vascular dementia. Neuroepidemiology 17(1):2–9

Small G 2002 What we need to know about age related memory loss. British Medical Journal 324:1502–1505

Snowdon D 1997 Aging and Alzheimer's disease: lessons from the Nun's study. Gerontologist 37(2):150–156

Wilkinson D 2001 Drugs for treatment of Alzheimer's disease. International Journal of Clinical Practice 55(2):129–134

World Health Organization 1992 ICD – 10. Classification of mental and behavioural disorders. Clinical descriptions and diagnostic guidelines. World Health Organization, Geneva

Further reading for carers or non-medical readers

Cayton H, Graham N, Warner J 2002 Dementia – Alzheimer's and other dementias at your fingertips, 2nd edn. Class Publishing, London

Cohen D, Eisdorfer C 2001 The loss of self. WW Norton, New York

Mace N, Rabins P, McHugh P 1999 The 36-hour day, 3rd edn. The Johns Hopkins University Press, Baltimore

Shenks D 2003 The forgetting. Understanding Alzheimer's disease: a biography of a disease. Harper Collins, London

Snowdon D 2002 Aging with grace. 4th Estate, London

Further reading

Ballard C, O'Brien J, James I, Swann A 2001 Dementia: management of behavioural and psychological symptoms. Oxford University Press, Oxford

Butler R, Pitt B 1998 Seminars in old age psychiatry. Gaskell, London

Chui E, Gustafson K, Ames D, Folstein M 1999 Cerebrovascular disease and dementia: pathology, neuropsychiatry and management. Martin Dunitz, London

Department of Health and the Welsh Office 1999 Mental Health Act 1983; Code of Practice. The Stationery Office, London

Hankey G 2002 Stroke. Your questions answered. Churchill Livingstone, Edinburgh

Hodges JR 1994 Cognitive assessment for physicians. Oxford Medical Publications, Oxford

Hodges JR (ed) 2001 Early onset dementia – a multidisciplinary approach. Oxford University Press, Oxford

Jacoby R, Oppenheimer C 2002 Psychiatry in the elderly, 3rd edn. Oxford Medical Publications, Oxford

The Law Society and the British Medical Association 1995 Assessment of mental capacity. Guidance for doctors and lawyers. British Medical Association, London

Lishman A 1998 Organic psychiatry, 3rd edn. Blackwell, Oxford

O'Brien J, Ames D, Burns A (eds) 2000 Dementia. Arnold, London

LIST OF PATIENT QUESTIONS

INDEX

*Numbers in **bold** refer to figures, tables and boxes*

D

T

X

Y

Z